Also by Carl Jones

Sharing Birth: A Father's Guide
to Giving Support During Labor

After the baby is born by Carl Jones

Photographs by Lyn Jones

Dodd, Mead & Company

New York

Copyright © 1986 by Carl Jones
All rights reserved
No part of this book may be reproduced in any form
without permission in writing from the publisher.
Published by Dodd, Mead & Company, Inc.
79 Madison Avenue, New York, N.Y. 10016
Distributed in Canada by
McClelland and Stewart Limited, Toronto
Manufactured in the United States of America
Designed by Kay Lee
First Edition

1 2 3 4 5 6 7 8 9 10

Library of Congress Cataloging-in-Publication Data

Jones, Carl.
    After the baby is born.

    Bibliography: p.
    Includes index.
    1. Childbirth. 2. Postnatal care. 3. Postpartum
depression—Prevention. 4. Exercise for women.
I. Title.
RG525.J66 1986   618.6   86-6219
ISBN 0-396-08789-2
ISBN 0-396-08790-6 (pbk.)

To my Mother

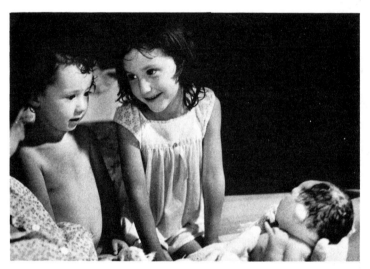

Photo by Stephanie Martin

Contents

❁   ❁   ❁

viii · *Contents*

Foreword

by *Mary Ellen Doherty*, R.N. C.N.M., M.S.
Certified Nurse-Midwife and
Childbirth Educator

Ever since its publication, I have recommended *Sharing Birth: A Father's Guide to Giving Support During Labor* as an invaluable aid to reducing the fear and pain of labor and achieving a positive birth experience.

Now Carl Jones has written *After the Baby Is Born*—an eminently practical, comprehensive, and concise post-partum guide. *After the Baby Is Born* encourages new parents to celebrate the joy of birth as it prepares them for the various changes that inevitably take place after birth.

There are more telephone calls to obstetrical offices from new mothers in the first few weeks after birth than at any other time. Couples are often given verbal post-partum instructions upon discharge from the hospital or birthing center. However, homecoming can be a time of excitement and chaos—a time when such verbal instructions are often forgotten. In *After the Baby Is Born*, all of the common questions and problems arising for new mothers are thoroughly covered. This sensitively written, illuminating book bridges the information gap and fulfills a long unmet need.

Carl Jones takes both parents on a marvelous journey, beginning with the first hour after birth. He leads mother and father through the sometimes wonderful, always challenging, occasionally exasperating, and never dull moments of their new lives as parents.

The mother learns precisely what is happening to her changing body, how to relieve the discomforts that often follow birth, how to regain her prepregnant figure, what exercises are most beneficial, and what remedies are most helpful in treating common postpartum problems.

When I discuss the postpartum period in my childbirth classes, I always involve the father. He can play a major supportive role, helping his partner cope with the various physiological and emotional changes that occur after giving birth.

After the Baby Is Born greatly emphasizes the father's supportive role and the importance of paternity leave. The father learns how to help his partner, how to minimize the "baby blues" if they occur, how his attitude can make the difference between breastfeeding success or failure, and how he can better relate to the transitions and changes in his own life.

After the Baby Is Born includes a wealth of practical suggestions to reduce stress, minimize apprehensions, and avoid problems at this very vulnerable time in one's life.

A childbirth educator and father himself, Carl Jones

combines a rare blend of experience, insight, and sensitivity. He is one of the few childbirth professionals and authors who understands equally well the needs of both women and men. I strongly recommend this book to expectant couples, postpartum couples, and childbirth professionals.

Foreword

by Martin Greenberg, M.D.

In my own work on paternal-infant attachment, I have found the early postpartum an important time in the new family's life. *After the Baby Is Born* tells the parents how to make the best of this life-transforming era.

Without doubt this is the best postpartum guide available and the only one to address the needs of *both* parents. Though the book is addressed to expectant and new mothers—discussing such topics as the mother's changing body and feelings and the special problems cesarean parents confront—*After the Baby Is Born* also clearly involves the father. It is a breath of fresh air to see the father's role discussed at a time when we hear increasing comments about the importance of women helping other women. While the supportive value of women in childbearing can't be denied, by focusing on women alone we can easily lose sight of and de-emphasize the man's crucial role.

Carl Jones emphasizes the need for paternity leave—something that I think is essential during the first few days after birth. No one can replace the father. He should be there at the beginning. In this way he will have an opportunity to feel a part of the unfolding family and share the joys and struggles that follow birth.

A childbirth educator and father himself, the author tells the new parents what he knows from personal experience—that they will feel not only joy after birth but other emotions, too. When our own son Jonathan was two weeks old, my wife Claudia and I went to a party to celebrate our new parenthood. Shortly after our arrival, the baby started crying. I attempted to still his cries to no avail. At that moment I felt like hiding in the corner of the room. I assumed that everyone was looking at me, judging me to be a failure. I wondered if I was really cut out to be a father.

Only later did I realize the universality of such emotions. Mothers and fathers experience a host of multi-faceted feelings when a child is born. Oftentimes insecurity, jealousy, and fear of responsibility may seem overwhelming. There may be times when both parents wish they could run away from the baby. *After the Baby Is Born* encourages readers to acknowledge such feelings and to allow themselves to experience the ambivalent emotions most new parents share.

This important book also covers the often under-emphasized but crucial things that parents wonder about but are perhaps afraid to ask in childbirth class—how the sexual relationship may change temporarily and what they can expect; how the father may feel about breastfeeding; and how both parents may be especially vulnerable and need each other's love.

In this book as in his former, *Sharing Birth: A Father's Guide to Giving Support During Labor*, Carl Jones once again proves that he has clearly been touched by the magic of the birth experience. He writes about birth as only he can—with tender insight and a special reverence born of his own love for the childbearing miracle. The nurturing glow of his words permeates this book and makes it a truly special guide.

Acknowledgments

Special thanks to the innumerable mothers and fathers who shared their births and birth stories with me.

Thanks also to those who have kindly read the manuscript and given me encouragement and suggestions: Mary Ellen Doherty, C.N.M. and childbirth educator in Sudbury, Massachusetts—an expert on the father's role through the childbearing season; Sloane Crawford, C.N.M. in private practice in Brookline, Massachusetts—a childbirth professional who leans toward the healing, rather than the clinical, dimensions of caring for the childbearing family; Martin Greenberg, M.D.—a pioneer in the burgeoning field of fathering literature; and David Stewart, Executive Director of the National Association for Parents and Professionals for Safe Alternatives in Childbirth (NAPSAC)—an organization that has done so much toward making positive changes in childbirth in America.

Above all, thanks to my wife Jan, who prepared the manuscript and who has been a continual source of inspiration.

After the baby is born

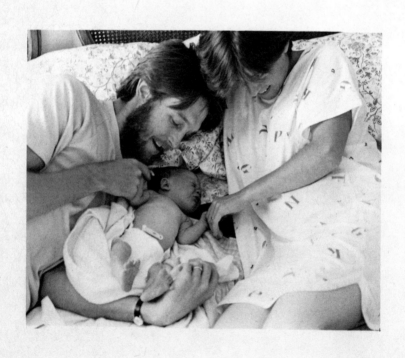

chapter one
· · · · · · · ·

The first few hours after birth

Suddenly labor is over—nature's most awesome miracle. The baby that has been so long within you is now in your arms. Physically, spiritually, emotionally, little compares with this experience.

One new mother said, "I couldn't stop crying, I was so happy." Another new mother summed up her feelings beautifully when after a long labor she lifted her child to her abdomen and shouted, "It's a baby! It's a baby! It's a baby!"

That first greeting is magical, unforgettable—one of life's peak events. As the mother's face brightens with elation, as the father's eyes well with tears, as the baby's eyes open to see the faces of his mother and his father for the first time in the dimly lit room, there is little to do but absorb the wonder of it.*

* I have chosen the pronoun "he" to avoid saying "he or she" every time the baby is mentioned.

Most new parents want to share their elation with everyone they know. They want to wake up their relatives, their friends, even if it is the middle of the night, and announce the wonderful news: A child is born. Life is forever changed.

The first six weeks after birth are referred to as the *postpartum period* (from Latin *post,* "after," and *partum,* "bearing" or the *puerperium* (from the Latin *puer,* "child," and *parere,* "to bear or bring forth"). During this time in the new mother's life several dramatic changes take place. Her body returns to its nonpregnant condition, her breasts adapt to nursing the child, and her emotions adjust to new motherhood.

The aftermath of the mother's pregnancy, the postpartum period, is sometimes referred to as the *fourth trimester.* (Pregnancy is divided into three periods of approximately three months each, called trimesters.) This culmination of the childbearing season is a life-altering era for both the baby and the parents.

THE FIRST HOUR

Of the six weeks following birth, the first hour is usually the most dramatic.

After the baby is born, you may feel elation, tremendous excitement, waves of love for your new child. You may be relieved that labor is over. And you may also be exhausted. Most new mothers experience a combination of all these feelings.

"When I held Christopher for the first time, I was in love," said Mary Ellen, a certified nurse-midwife, after the birth of her first child. "I explored him with my hands and announced to everyone that he was a boy."

Martin, a new father, said, "It was a wonderful experience! Just being with Jonathan for the hour before they took him to be weighed and so forth made the three of us very close. Jonathan had come to join Sheila and me together very strongly."

Overwhelming emotion followed our own first birth. In my excitement I forgot to take the photographs I promised myself I would include in the family album, to be forever cherished. (A good reason it is wise to leave birth photography to a friend or relative!) Meanwhile, my wife Jan was sitting on the bed breastfeeding our newborn son Carl in utter ecstasy, her face radiant.

Yolana and Chris gave birth at home. Chris caught the baby as Yolana cried, "It's out! It's out! I have a baby!"

Chris recalls the moment as especially magical. "Yolana's voice never sounded the same before and never sounded the same again." Afterward the mother said, "I can't remember whether we spent one hour or five together, I was so caught up with the baby."

Following the birth of their 9 lb. 14 oz. son Alex, Linda and her husband, Matthew, shared the same ecstatic emotion. "Beautiful!" the mother exclaimed. The intensity of Linda's joy was heightened by the fact that she had longed for a vaginal birth after having given birth to triplets by cesarean section four years before.

Birth, however, is not always followed by feelings of joy or waves of love. Disappointment, frustration, or simple exhaustion are perfectly normal, especially if things haven't gone as planned or there has been a very long labor. "I was utterly wiped out after Kristen was born," one new mother said. "All I wanted to do was be left alone to sleep."

There is no particular way you *should* feel. There are a variety of reasons why new mothers feel and react differently after birth. Among the factors that influence your immediate after-birth reaction are: the length of your labor; the birthing environment; your health care during labor and birth; whether or not you have had obstetrical medication; whether or not you have had an episiotomy (a surgical incision to enlarge the birth outlet as the baby's head is born) and must wait for it to be stitched; your relationship with your partner; and, of course, the health of your baby.

A Sensitive Time

Doctors Klaus and Kennel, in their book *Maternal Infant Bonding*,[1] have called attention to the fact that the first hour or so following birth is a sensitive period. This is usually characterized by a period of high energy for the mother, father, and baby if they have experienced a natural birth. The mother "takes in" and receives her child. If born naturally, the baby is generally exceptionally alert for an hour or so before sleeping deeply for another three or four hours. He also is in a "taking in" phase. This vitally important phase in the childbearing drama begins the ongoing process of parental-infant attachment.

Close contact during this sensitive period facilitates this attachment, known as "bonding." Studies have shown that mothers who have had prolonged contact with their infants shortly after birth demonstrate greater affection and attachment for their babies later on. On the other hand, research has also shown that there is a greater percentage of neglect, abuse, and failure to thrive among infants who are separated from their parents shortly after birth.[2, 3]

There are many variations in the way new mothers behave when the baby is born. There is enough similarity, though, to have led some health professionals to consider early maternal behavior "species specific"—that is, the members of any one given species pretty much follow the same basic pattern. The way human mothers touch and explore their babies is said to follow a general pattern: first exploring the baby's head and extremities with her fingertips, then caressing the trunk with her open palm, and finally enfolding the baby in her arms.

Most fathers who attend birth also want to participate actively in the attachment process. When Johanna and Steve's first child, Sarah, was born in a hospital birthing room, she had barely a minute at Johanna's breast before the ecstatic father asked to hold her. Though it was his first child, Steve held Sarah as if he had had many children before. For the next half hour he stared into her eyes, totally caught up in the magic that so often follows birth. Finally he looked up at Johanna. "Aren't you glad you birthed naturally?" The mother said she was.

Being an active participant in the childbearing miracle makes the transition to parenthood smoother for both mother and father.

Julia was born in a hospital birthing room. After the physician assisted with the birth of the baby's head (that part of delivery most in need of expert supervision), the mother, Carolyn, and her husband, Jim, completed the birth themselves. Carolyn reached down and lifted her child toward her, one hand under each of the baby's arms, while Jim supported the baby's back with his hand. Still half inside her mother's body, Julia opened her eyes. The expression on Carolyn's face during this moment of eye contact was unforgettable. Tears streamed down her cheeks and over her broad, smiling mouth. She lifted her baby immediately to her breast. Shortly afterward, Jim cut the cord.

Many parents like to be the first to touch their child, to "catch" the baby themselves as it is born (though it is always wise to have a competent caregiver present at birth). But whether or not you catch your own baby, as Carolyn and Jim did, taking an active role in birth to the degree that you both feel comfortable will make a difference. Being fully involved emotionally, and knowing that you are in charge of the way you give birth, enables you to feel more fully involved with your new role afterward. This is largely because having taken an active part, you tend to view birth as a family affair—a part of your own natural parenting ability—rather than as a medical procedure.

Though spending the first hour or so after birth together is important, it is not essential for an optimum relationship with your child. Needless to say, love cannot be reduced to a series of invariable biological patterns. If you are not able to enjoy the first postnatal hour with your baby, don't feel guilty. You will still develop parent-infant attachment. The love you feel for your child and the love your child feels for you is ongoing.

After an exhausting four-day labor, Kim and Rob's plans for a natural birth without medical intervention were abruptly changed. Kim was given the hormonal solution Pitocin to augment the labor contractions, which, in Kim's case, were not dilating the cervix. She was later moved from the birthing room (where she had planned to give birth) to the delivery room as a result of meconium staining in the amniotic waters. (Meconium is the baby's first stool. Its release before birth is a sign of possible fetal distress.) Flat on her back and unable to participate, she found the delivery quite frightening.

"After the birth of Caitlyn," she recalls, "they took her away to suction mucus from her nose and throat. Later, when they brought her to me wrapped in a receiving blanket, with only her little pink face showing, I didn't feel love for her right away. I was angry at myself and then started to cry. The nurse asked me if I wanted to hold her or if she should take her to the nursery. I couldn't comfortably hold her on the narrow table while being stitched, so I chose the nursery. Almost immediately I felt I was betraying her. 'Go with her,' I told my husband, Rob. I felt that one of us should be with her."

Afterward, Kim and Rob shared intense love for their child. Rob says, "Caitlyn was so much fun. She was rarely out of our arms for six weeks."

You can have a fulfilling, rewarding postpartum period even if there are complications. New mothers recovering from cesarean surgery, for example, are just as able to nurse and enjoy the time after birth with their baby as those who have delivered vaginally—though they perhaps feel more uncomfortable during the early days.

The following basic suggestions will insure making the most of the time shortly following birth.

Remain with your child for at least the first hour after birth. The ideal place for the baby during this precious hour is in your arms, held skin to skin against your body. A receiving blanket and a hat on the baby's head will provide sufficient warmth. While you hold your child, he will grasp a finger or a lock of hair tightly in his tiny hand if you make either available to him.

Be sure the room is dimly lit. After birth, your baby will open his eyes and look around. If it is very sunny, the shades should be drawn so the light won't hurt the baby's sensitive eyes.

For the newborn, leaving the womb is probably like stepping out of a dark room into the sunny outdoors after a snowstorm. At first, the blinding light hurts. It takes time to adjust. The baby has spent months in relative darkness. If the room is dimly lit the baby will be able to see. He can best see and recognize objects that are close to his face—in fact, just the distance he will be from your face when you hold him to your breast.

The baby may have spots of *vernix caseosa*, a white creamy substance on the skin, especially around the creases of the armpits and groin. This luxurious-feeling substance protected the baby's skin while in the uterus. Rather than removing it, rub it into the skin. If there is an excessive amount, it can be used later as a rich, emollient skin cream.

Some new parents wish to give the baby a Leboyer-style bath, immersing him in a small basin of warm water. Babies seem to find this particularly relaxing. It probably lessens the trauma of being born in the noisy and often impersonal environment of a large hospital. But there is no substitute for holding your baby skin to skin in peaceful, supportive surroundings.

Avoid interruption. Be sure all medical procedures, including weighing and measuring the baby, are delayed for an hour or two after birth (unless there is an emergency). Avoid especially the use of prophylactic eye drops (to prevent gonococcal-caused blindness) until *after* the first hour. Eye drops may sting and/or blur the baby's vision, preventing that wonderful eye contact that otherwise follows normal birth.

If the birth is normal, and you and your baby are healthy, medical procedures can easily be postponed. Then, when you are ready, the baby can be examined, weighed, and measured.

If there is an emergency and the baby must be taken to an intensive care unit immediately after birth, accompany your child. If you have had a cesarean or are having an episiotomy stitched, and the baby must be taken to a special care nursery, your partner can accompany the baby there and share his first actions with you later.

After Anne's second child was born, the baby was immediately removed to a nursery because her respiration and heart rate were low and her color poor. "I was so upset that they had to take me to the baby," Anne recalls. "Since I had no strength in my legs, they took me to her via wheelchair." Asking to, or if necessary insisting upon, accompanying your baby, as this new mother did, is a perfectly reasonable request.

In a few hospitals, the importance of a natural after-birth follow-up is not yet recognized. Immediately or shortly after birth, babies are routinely taken to an infant warmer, usually on the other side of the room from their mother, where the newborn exam or medical procedures take place. Or, after mother and baby have spent only a few minutes together, the baby is removed to a central nursery to be weighed and measured.

Such practices hinder a normal and vital process. They impair the natural response of both parents and child, as well as increase anxiety and after-birth trauma. They should therefore be avoided.

If your hospital doesn't routinely encourage prolonged maternal-infant contact after birth, ask to be allowed to remain with your baby without interruption. If necessary, insist. Don't feel that you are demanding a special favor. It is your baby, not the hospital's.

Actually, when you think about it, removing an infant from its mother to an artificial infant warmer for routine procedures is a rather bizarre custom. No animal breeder would do such an odd thing, because animal breeders recognize the negative effects maternal-infant separation have on both mother and offspring. Why, then, is maternal-infant separation a common practice with humans, who have a more highly developed nervous system and are more sensitive than animals?

The practice originated in the era when many women were unconscious during delivery and were unable to interact with their babies right after birth. Though the practice of separating mother and baby is falling by the wayside, it still survives in a few hospitals that have not yet developed a more humanistic approach to birth.

You may have to be assertive to get what you want in some hospitals. It is best for your partner to interface with the staff, as you will probably be too fatigued. As one new mother said: "Jerry made a positive nuisance of himself. The nurses couldn't stand him because he wouldn't allow anything to be done unless we first approved." Ideally, of course, it is better to avoid negative confrontation of any kind by having chosen a birth place conducive to beginning a new family.

Offer the baby the breast immediately after birth. It is

wise to do this whether or not you plan to breastfeed, for your benefit as well as the baby's.

For you. Nursing immediately following birth facilitates third-stage labor (the delivery of the placenta). Nature designed a delicate interrelationship between immediate breastfeeding and the conclusion of labor. When the baby sucks the breast, the pituitary gland releases the hormone oxytocin, which causes the uterus to contract and deliver the placenta. After the placenta is delivered, oxytocin helps keep the uterine muscles clamped tightly around the open blood vessels at the placental site, preventing postpartum hemorrhage. Finally, immediate nursing is the best way for you and your newborn to snuggle and be close.

For your baby. The premilk substance called *colostrum*, secreted by the breasts until the milk "comes in" about the third postpartum day, is rich in many of your baby's essential needs. Among these are vitamins, nutrients, and fluids the baby needs to clear excess mucus from his mouth and throat. Colostrum also contains antibodies to many viral and bacterial diseases, helping to prevent infections, particularly of the intestinal tract. Also, while sucking at the breast, the baby is close to you and feels secure.

Rhona, a first-time mother who originally planned to bottle-feed, said, "I didn't want to be tied down nursing a baby for several months. But holding Ian at my breast just for those first few minutes changed my mind." Like Rhona, other new mothers who planned to bottle-feed have found that this initial nursing experience reversed their decision.

The baby may not take the breast as soon as it is offered. Some babies have a little difficulty getting started, or just don't seem to be interested at first, while others take the nipple voraciously.

Be sure both parents are involved.   The father also can remove his shirt and hold the infant skin to skin shortly after birth. Or, he can get in bed with the mother and baby and share in the cuddling. Holding the baby to his chest and sharing eye contact is an intense experience for most fathers.

After the birth of his daughter, Jamie, one new father said, "Looking into her eyes for the first time was the height of the whole miraculous event. It seemed even more of a miracle than the birth itself."

Involve your other children.   Birth is a family affair affecting every family member—especially your other children. Siblings should visit with the baby shortly after birth (if they have not attended the birth), *not* several days later. They should see the infant face to face, not merely through the glass window of a nursery, and they should touch the baby. Check with your hospital to be sure this is encouraged *before* planning to birth there. A few hospitals restrict sibling visitation.

The best birthing and immediate postpartum environment is a place where you feel safe, comfortable, and supported emotionally. A peaceful, supportive birth place where you are free to labor in whatever position is comfortable, invite whomever you wish to share your birth, and so forth, influences the way you labor and how you feel after birth. You are bound to be more relaxed in a comfortable birthing environment, more able to respond to labor and to your newborn appropriately.

Next to home, the childbearing center often provides the most comfortable place to give birth and begin a new family. One of my associate childbirth instructors refers to childbearing centers as "half-way steps between home and hospital."

Shirley, a mother of three, gave birth to her first two children at a birthing center. The third was born in a hospital. Having moved to a new home during her third pregnancy, the mother recalls, "We opted for the hospital because it was so close and convenient.

"During my first two pregnancies," Shirley continues, "I went for prenatal exams to the place where I was going to have my baby. I became familiar with the birthing center, comfortable. I also met everyone who might be attending my labor.

"After my second birth, the baby never left me for a minute. My husband, Conrad, lay next to me on a double bed and we slept with the baby."

After the third birth, Conrad remarked, "Everything seemed much more natural for the first two births. I wish we had gone to a birthing center for the third."

"In retrospect," Shirley adds, "I now understand the difference and would never make that choice again.

"When I went to the hospital for the third birth, I walked in and was immediately faced with strangers. The baby was swept away from me fifteen minutes after birth. There was supposed to be a lot of skin contact. But we didn't share that. They gave me my baby swaddled.

"Every step of the way throughout my postpartum stay, it was a tug of war. It seemed that I was continually struggling to have the baby with me while the nurses were struggling to get the baby into the nursery.

"The difference between the birth center and the hospital was that in the hospital I didn't have as much control over my body or my baby."

Thanks to an emerging humanistic maternity care, hospitals are changing and becoming better environments to begin a family. However, disappointments such as Shirley's are by no means uncommon.

If planning a hospital birth, it is best to avoid a clinical atmosphere or an institution with rigid policies. Birthing rooms, backed by a staff that practices noninterventive care, are more conducive to getting to know your child than the more sterile-looking delivery room. The birthing room provides the more agreeable place to begin a family. And beds are always more comfortable than narrow delivery tables, giving you the freedom to move around as you wish, and allowing the father to sit or lie snuggling with the newborn at your side.

If, however, you do give birth in less than perfect surroundings, you can still have a positive experience. After the birth of her 8 lb. 2 oz. daughter, Johanna, a first-time mother, said, "We planned to use the birthing room. But when my husband, Justin, and I arrived at the hospital, the birthing room was occupied. We were moved to a delivery room just before birth. Though I was at first upset that we were not allowed to remain in the labor room, we were so overwhelmed when Karla was born that it no longer mattered where we were. I gave birth on the same bed where I labored rather than moving to the delivery table. The room was dimly lit throughout and we were permitted to remain together there as long as we wanted."

Remaining in a delivery room after birth is not always possible in a busy hospital. But wherever you are, the important thing is that you, your partner, and your baby remain together.

At birth, you and your child both experience a transition to a new life. The first hour ushers your baby into life outside the womb, as it ushers you and your partner into parenthood. Remaining together during this time is the way to make sure your new life together has the best possible beginning.

After the first hour, it is wise for you, your partner, and your baby to continue being together, avoiding unnecessary interruptions. You can arrange that the newborn exam take place in your immediate presence (not across the room). In some hospitals, you can remain in the same room where you have given birth, rather than moving to a separate recovery or postpartum room, eliminating an unnecessary change in environment.

Whether birth takes place in a hospital or a childbearing center, ideally the three of you can remain together until discharge. Many hospitals and most childbearing centers arrange for discharge of mother and infant two to twenty-four hours after birth if both are in good health. Then you can continue your transition to new parenthood at home.

ROOMING-IN

If you do have to stay in the hospital, rooming-in (you and your baby remaining in the same room throughout your postpartum stay) is an option available at most hospitals. Rooming-in is the best way to facilitate breastfeeding and enhance the natural maternal-infant relationship after birth.

If you choose to room-in, you need not have your baby with you every minute. A nurse will take the baby to the nursery if you wish. A similar option is modified rooming-in, in which case the baby is with you for part of the time.

Don't expect to enjoy every minute of rooming-in. There is nothing abnormal if you find it trying at times—especially at 2 A.M. when the baby is crying.

Choose a hospital where your partner can remain with you, twenty-four hours a day, if possible. In some hospitals the father also can room-in, sleeping with his partner on a double bed. This way the family is off to the best start with the least amount of trauma resulting from separation during a particularly sensitive time.

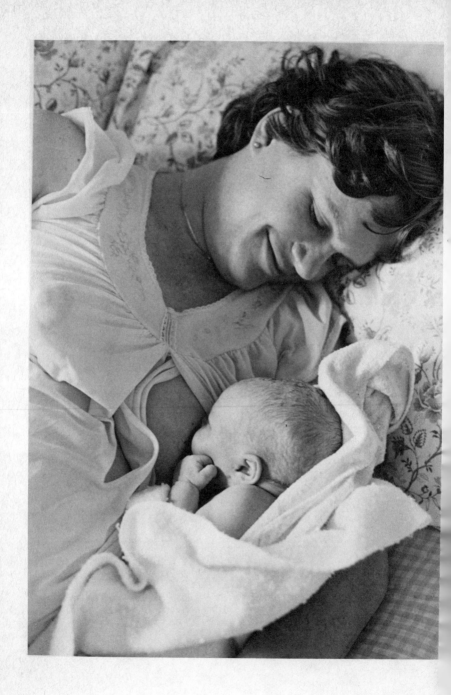

chapter two
· · · · · · · ·

Your changing body

The miracle of birth triggers in many a deep respect and sense of wonder for the power of a woman's body. It is truly amazing that the uterus, where the baby has grown and developed for nine calendar months, is able to contract rhythmically and open the cervical opening, little by little, to permit a child to pass from his cushioned, watery home to the world outside. It is incredible that the narrow birth canal can stretch to give passage to a baby whose head is as large as a grapefruit, and still return to its former shape. The marvelous changes associated with childbearing don't end with labor. From the moment of birth, the body continues to undergo amazing transformations.

Birth is a perfectly normal event, not an illness from which you recover. Unless you've had cesarean surgery or other complications, getting back into shape will take place rapidly and efficiently. After all, nature designed mothers to be able to give birth and immediately begin caring for their babies.

The first postpartum hour, beginning with the birth of the placenta, is often referred to as the "fourth stage of labor." Though not really part of labor, it is a critical part of the postpartum recovery process. Your caregiver* will examine the placenta and the umbilical cord, taking a sample of cord blood. Your perineum† will be examined. If you have torn it, or had an episiotomy, it will be sutured at this time. The uterus will also be palpated with a hand on the abdomen to make sure it is properly contracted and to rule out the possibility of hemorrhage.

THE NEED FOR REST

As long as you get plenty of rest and take it easy, you don't have to stay in bed during waking hours after a natural birth unless you want to. In fact, you don't even have to give birth in bed. Some women prefer squatting on the floor. Many hospitals now have birthing chairs or simply bean bag chairs. After birth you can be up and about whenever you feel like it. Let your body be your guide about when to get up and how much to do at first.

Be sure to have assistance the first time out of bed

---

* The term "caregiver" is used throughout this book to indicate any person who provides health care during pregnancy, labor, and the postpartum period. The caregiver may be a midwife, obstetrician, family practitioner, naturopath, chiropractor, and so forth.

† "Perineum," like "crotch," is a confusing and somewhat vague term. Deriving from two Greek words for "around" and "to empty" or "to defecate," perineum has more than one meaning. It describes the external area roughly corresponding to the outlet of the pelvis surrounding the urinary, genital, and anal openings. Perineum also refers to the area between the vagina (or in the male, the scrotum) and the anus.

until you are sure there is no dizziness, lightheadedness, weakness in the knees, or a feeling that you might faint or fall. A nurse or your caregiver will help you in the hospital or childbearing center. Your partner can help you if you give birth at home.

Many healthy new mothers are surprised by how tired they feel. "I never expected to feel so tired and run down," said Mandy a month after her first child was born. "There were so many things I wanted to do immediately, but couldn't." Kathy Kangas, childbirth educator and founder of Birth Unlimited in Millbury, Massachusetts, says, "A lot of my students expect to have a baby and feel just as good as they did before they got pregnant. But they soon discover that recovery takes time."

If you've had more than one baby, you may feel different after each birth. "I was so wide awake and excited that I couldn't sleep after the birth of Landon," Kathy Kangas continues. "But when Annsie was born, I was exhausted."

Not all women experience tiredness. My own wife, Jan, was up and about within an hour or so after our second son, Paul, was born. Later that day we took a short walk in the country—a rather brisk walk with sub-zero wind on our faces. We kept expecting a great wave of exhaustion—primarily because all the books insist that postpartum women feel tired! But there was no excessive tiredness that day, or in the weeks that followed. We attribute Jan's vitality and her rapid postpartum recovery largely to a wholly natural birth preceded by a well-balanced diet and regular mountain hiking throughout pregnancy.

However you feel after birth—full of vitality or exhausted—you should get plenty of rest. Don't try to resume immediately your ordinary daily activities beyond baby care. Dramatic physical changes take place during the first postpartum weeks. The simple basics—rest, relaxation, and walking in the fresh air—will contribute to a rapid postpartum recovery, while help around the home will make life immeasurably smoother.

Rest after the baby comes is essential for both physical and emotional well-being. Overactivity may lead to fatigue, interfere with the postpartum recovery process, and possibly predispose the mother to complications.

Generally speaking, home is the best place for a new mother and father to get much needed rest after birth (unless there are medical complications). Hospitals are rarely restful. As one childbirth educator put it: "If you insist on rest-time away from home after the baby is born, go to a motel or an inn. The industry that caters to guests is far better at providing rest and relaxation than a hospital."

POSTPARTUM WEIGHT LOSS

Birth is the only time in your life when you lose twelve to fifteen pounds in a single day! When the baby (average weight seven and a half pounds), the placenta (two pounds), and the amniotic fluid (one and a half pounds) are delivered, inches immediately drop from your abdomen. The belly, however, will probably still remain floppy for several weeks.

Another five pounds will probably be lost during the first postpartum weeks through urine and heavy perspiration. *Diuresis*, an increased excretion of urine, is normal after childbirth, helping to eliminate fluids retained during pregnancy.

Later, you will probably lose additional weight as the uterus shrinks. The enlarged uterus alone is responsible for two extra pounds.

You should not expect to return to your prepregnancy weight until the fourth or sixth postpartum month, though you may do so sooner. It is unwise to begin a strict diet while nursing, as your body needs additional calories, protein, and nutrients to produce milk, but cutting down on empty calories will certainly help.

The same areas most stressed during pregnancy—the abdominal region, back, reproductive organs, and pelvic-floor muscles—are those most in need of conditioning after birth. Regular exercise, beginning as soon as possible after birth, will help you regain your prepregnant shape, strengthen your abdomen, and tone the pelvic floor, as well as prevent back problems and minor complications such as constipation and urinary incontinence. This will be discussed in more detail in Chapter 5.

THE REPRODUCTIVE ORGANS

The Uterus

The earliest and most dramatic postpartum change takes place in the uterus. Marked progressive changes in the size, weight, and position of this amazing organ begin shortly following birth. This process by which the uterus returns to its almost original size and pear shape is called *involution* (like evolution in reverse).

During pregnancy, the uterus grows to about eleven times its prepregnant weight and becomes large enough to hold 500 times its former capacity. Following birth, the now empty uterus weighs over two pounds, a week later one pound, and in two weeks about twelve ounces. When involution is complete, it weighs about two ounces.

Immediately after the placenta is delivered, the baby's former home, no longer needed, collapses into a tight mass. At this time the uterus should be midway between the navel and the pubic bone, where it feels quite hard, like a ball of muscle. A nurse or your caregiver will check the uterus to make sure it remains hard, indicating that the muscles are clamped tightly around the blood vessels at the placental site. Should the uterus become soft and boggy, your caregiver or a nurse will massage it until it becomes firm.

A relaxed uterus (*uterine atony*) is the major cause of excessive bleeding in the immediate postpartum period. Though uncommon, uterine atony may be the result of several factors, including: a uterus overdistended as a result of multiple babies or excessive amniotic fluid; an unusually long labor; previous uterine surgery (not including cesarean surgery); uterine fibroids; and maternal diseases such as pre-eclampsia, anemia, and so forth.

With your caregiver's guidance, you can massage the uterus yourself if you wish. With one hand, use a firm circular motion just below the navel. Stop massaging once the uterus becomes firm. Overmassaging can cause a firm uterus once again to become boggy.

Later, the uterus actually rises again in the abdomen, like a yeast bread, and reaches the navel. Within about twelve hours, the top of the uterus can be felt a little above the navel.

You can follow the progress of uterine involution for about ten days after birth, as the uterus sinks in the abdominal cavity like a slowly deflating balloon one fingerwidth or so (about one-half inch) a day. By the tenth day, the uterus can no longer be felt above the pubic bone except via bimanual exam (one finger in the vagina against the cervix, the other hand above the pubic bone). Involution usually progresses more efficiently in women who nurse their babies.

As the uterus alternately relaxes and contracts, you may experience *afterpains* (also called *after-birth pains*), mild to severe laborlike cramps. Afterpains are more pronounced in women who have given birth before, and may persist for a few days. Relieving the discomfort is discussed in Chapter 3.

As the uterus involutes, the muscle cells actually become smaller. Material from the uterine walls is broken down, absorbed, and eliminated both through the urine and by means of a vaginal discharge called *lochia* (from the Greek word for "childbirth").

Before pregnancy, the uterus had been shedding the outer layer of the *endometrium,* the specialized lining of the uterus, every month during menstruation, as a deciduous tree sheds its leaves. In fact, this resemblance to leaf-shedding trees has earned the name *decidua* (from Latin, "to fall away") for this rich outer portion of the endometrium. During pregnancy, the decidua becomes quite thick and provides the fertile bed in which the egg implants. Here the placenta begins to develop and burrow into the uterine lining with projections much like the roots of a tree.

After birth, the decidua, no longer needed, is shed. This is a primary constituent of lochia. The regeneration of the endometrium is usually accomplished by the fifth or sixth week.

When involution is complete, the uterus will remain slightly larger than it was before pregnancy. But this is nothing you will be able to notice.

Lochia, a discharge made up of uterine lining cast off during the early postpartum period, blood, and vaginal secretions, begins like a heavy menstrual flow and then tapers off. For the first three days after birth, lochia consists primarily of blood and is red. This is called *lochia rubra*. During this time, some of the lochia may be expelled in the form of clots. After the third day the discharge becomes more pink or brown and is also somewhat watery. It is then called *lochia serosa* (from the Latin for "watery fluid" or "serum"). Finally, about ten days after birth, lochia is almost colorless or yellowish, at which time it is called *lochia alba*. Lochia gradually tapers off, usually within a week, but it may last up to six weeks. This varies from mother to mother.

You may notice an increase in the amount of lochia after getting up from a lying position as a result of pooling in the vagina. Lochia may also be more reddish after physical activity.

A return of blood-tinged lochia after the discharge has faded usually indicates you are overdoing it. Take it easy. Bright red bleeding after the fourth postbirth day, however, should be reported to your caregiver without delay. It may indicate hemorrhage, possibly caused by retained placental fragments.

You will have to use sanitary napkins for a week or so, perhaps longer. Do not use tampons, as they increase the possibility of infection. Change the sanitary pads every four to six hours and each time you urinate or defecate. Be sure the pad is on securely. When removing the pad, do so from front to back to avoid infecting the area with anal bacteria. Wearing cotton pants that breathe and stay dry discourages infections and itching.

The normal odor of lochia is "fleshy," like that of menstrual blood. It may smell stronger if mixed with perspiration, but it should not have an offensive odor.

WARNING

- Persistent release of clots or persistent red lochia may be caused by retained placental fragments.
- Offensive odor may indicate infection.
- Scant lochia during the first few days may indicate that uterine involution is not progressing properly.
- Heavy lochia (soaking more than one large pad within one-half hour) that does not diminish with rest, or episodes of brisk painless bleeding, may indicate that the placental site is not recovering properly.

Any of the above conditions should be referred to your caregiver without delay.

If you have any concern that you are losing too much blood, consult your caregiver. Excessive bleeding sometimes results from lacerations to the vagina and cervix. Occasionally, hemorrhage is caused by retained placental fragments, sometimes as long as a week or two after birth.

Actual menstrual periods usually re-establish themselves within eight weeks in a nonnursing mother, and in a nursing mother anytime between two and eighteen months, with an average of five to six months. Sometimes a nursing mother may not begin menstruating until the baby is partially or completely weaned.

Your first menstrual flow may be heavier than usual.

The Cervix
The cervix, the neck of the uterus that protrudes into the vagina, rapidly assumes its nonpregnant state.

During pregnancy, the cervix changes in consistency from that of a hard lump of muscle to something as soft as an earlobe. The dimple-shaped cervical opening, called the external *os* (from the Latin word for "mouth" or "opening"), may *dilate* (open) one, two, or more centimeters before labor begins. During labor, of course, the cervix dilates sufficiently to give the baby passage.

After birth, the cervix is left floppy and still stretchable for a while. It will permit the passage of about two finger-breadths ten or twelve hours later. But within eighteen hours the cervix will once again become firm. By the end of the first week, the cervix just about reaches its nonpregnant state. The os, however, is no longer shaped like a circle, as it was before pregnancy, but remains a transverse slit.

The Vagina
In the poetry of India and China, the vagina has often been compared to a flower. This is an especially appropriate image for the birth canal during childbearing, when this marvelous organ really does appear to open like a flower.

After having stretched to form a gateway for the birth

of your baby, the vagina may be left gaping open for a day or two. It may also feel slack for a couple of weeks after birth. But the vagina will soon return to nearly its prepregnant state. "The Blossom" exercise in Chapter 5 will help regain vaginal tone.

During pregnancy, the vagina's velvety walls change from pink to violet colored as a result of additional blood supply. After birth they will once again turn pink. The labia will remain a little darker and somewhat more flaccid.

Possible tears (or an incision) will heal by the end of the postpartum period. Relieving perineal discomfort is discussed in Chapter 4.

The Pelvic-Floor Muscles

A sheet of pelvic floor muscle slung from the pubic bone in front to the *coccyx* (tail bone) in back supports the uterus and its contents much like a hammock. Known as the *pubococcygeal muscle*, this controls the three openings: vagina, urethra, and anus.

The pelvic floor's musculature is considerably stretched when the baby is born. After birth, it is left loose and sagging. Though the effects of this are not visible, a weakened pelvic floor can later result in decreased vaginal tone, urinary incontinence, and other gynecological problems.

Exercising the pelvic floor will help the musculature resume its former condition, restore vaginal tone, and help prevent other problems.

Even with a cesarean birth, the muscles are stretched as a result of the additional weight of the uterus and its contents, and the effects of hormones, so you should still exercise the pelvic floor.

The Abdomen

During pregnancy, the abdomen expands considerably to accommodate the growing baby and enlarging uterus. The abdominal muscles actually double in length by the time the baby is born. Though your waistline will immediately lose several inches at birth, the belly will probably be left looking flabby. One new mother said, "After I had the baby, my stomach rippled and flopped all over the place like a waterbed every time I touched it."

If you exercise regularly, the abdomen will probably begin to resume its prepregnant shape by the end of the six postpartum weeks. Of course, this depends on your prepregnant condition and how much weight you gained during pregnancy.

The *abdominal recti*, a pair of muscles that run down either side of the abdomen in twin sheets, have a tendency to separate like a broken zipper during pregnancy and to remain slightly separated afterward. Some degree of separation, known as *diastasis recti*, is quite common and nothing to be worried about. If the separation is wide enough, however, it can lead to a flabby belly, back problems, and more difficult subsequent pregnancies. How to check for the degree of separation and correct this condition is discussed in Chapter 5.

Other Changes

There is considerable blood loss with the delivery of the placenta. The loss is greater if you have had an episiotomy or a large tear. During pregnancy, however, the total blood volume has increased over 30 percent and you can well tolerate the loss. Your caregiver will watch for excessive loss during the first few hours after birth. Afterward, you should bear in mind that red lochia discharge should not soak more than one large pad within one half hour.

It is perfectly normal for the new mother to go without a bowel movement for two or three days after birth. Several factors may contribute to this delay: decreased muscle tone in the intestines; prelabor diarrhea that cleared the bowels; lack of food during labor; dehydration; and perineal tenderness as a result of tearing, an episiotomy, and/or hemorrhoids. Relieving constipation (if you fail to have a bowel movement after three to five postpartum days) and the discomfort of hemorrhoids are discussed in Chapter 4.

Your temperature may be as high as 100.4° F during the first twenty-four hours after birth as a result of the dehydrating effects of labor. A low-grade fever (100° F) after this time may be the result of a minor problem or may accompany breast engorgement.

If your temperature rises *after* the first twenty-four hours and recurs or persists for two days, it may indicate infection. Should fever develop, drink plenty of fluids and consult your caregiver without delay.

Changes in skin pigmentation acquired during pregnancy will usually disappear after the baby is born. The increased pigmentation of the breasts and abdomen, however, will not disappear entirely, though it will fade somewhat.

Stretch marks, pink or reddish streaks covering the sides of the abdomen and sometimes the inner and outer thighs, will fade. They take on a silvery white appearance but don't disappear entirely.

THE BREASTS

Though we know enough today about the composition of breast milk to realize that it is the ideal food for babies, milk production is still largely a mystery.

Breast changes in preparation for lactation begin early on and continue throughout pregnancy. Fullness, heightened sensitivity, tingling, and heaviness of the breasts occur in the first trimester. Veins become more noticeable, the nipples more erect, and the *areola*, the pigmented area around the nipple, darker. Glands of Montgomery, little bumps in the areola that secrete material to lubricate and protect the nipple, become more prominent by the first or second month.

Meanwhile, the milk-secreting and milk-duct system develops. Within each breast are fifteen to twenty ducts, little milk-bearing canals, each connecting the nipple to the lobes, where the milk is made. The lobes are like tiny clusters of grapes. Each consists of smaller lobules, which are made up of little sacs called *alveoli,* lined with milk-secreting cells. Near the lobes the ducts (corresponding to the stem of the grape cluster) branch out to the different lobules. Underneath the areola the ducts widen into milk sinuses (lactiferous sinuses). When the baby sucks the nipple, actually compressing the milk sinuses under the areola with his lips, gum, and tongue, he forces the milk out of the many openings of the nipple into his mouth.

During pregnancy, hormones manufactured by the placenta contribute to changes in the glandular breast tissue. The milk-bearing ducts elongate and branch out. The alveoli sacs further develop and begin to produce milk. By the fifth or sixth month of pregnancy, milk is in the breasts. However, it isn't secreted until after the placenta is delivered. (The size of the breasts has nothing to do with the ability to nurse successfully. Breast size is related to the amount of fatty tissue, not the glandular, milk-producing tissue.)

After birth, the breasts first secrete colostrum, the previously mentioned, high-protein, yellowish premilk substance very important for the baby's health. About the second or third day the milk "comes in." At this time the breasts may become swollen and engorged for twenty-four to forty-eight hours, whether or not you are nursing. Breast engorgement is less likely if the mother begins nursing immediately after birth and nurses "on demand"—that is, whenever the baby wants milk. Relieving engorgement is discussed further in Chapter 4.

When the milk is removed from the breasts, whether via the baby's sucking or manually expressed, more milk is produced. The supply eventually adjusts to the demand as you and your baby develop a nursing pattern. This occurs most efficiently when you nurse on demand.

If your baby is sick or premature and must stay in the hospital, you can express and store breast milk to bring to him there.

Two basic processes are involved in nursing: the baby's sucking and the *let-down reflex*, that is, the milk secretion or milk ejection reflex. Though it may seem as if the baby removes the milk from the breasts by sucking, this is only part of the nursing process. By sucking, the baby gets only the milk in the milk sinuses under the areola.

The let-down reflex, a term borrowed from dairymen who speak of cows "letting down" the milk, causes the milk sinuses to fill as the baby empties them.

Helen Varney, author of *Nurse-Midwifery*, describes

this process as "an exquisite blend of neurological, hormonal, and psychological factors in which the latter can totally inhibit and frustrate the others and also frustrate the baby and mother."[1] When the baby sucks the breast, the hormone oxytocin is released by the pituitary gland (in the brain), causing cells surrounding the alveoli and milk-bearing ducts to contract, thus pushing the milk through the ducts to the milk sinuses under the nipple. The milk may leak or even spray when it is let down. Many new mothers find the let-down triggered and the breasts leaking even before the baby sucks, when he cries, or even when they think about the baby.

A relaxed, unhurried attitude and emotionally supportive surroundings facilitate successful nursing. Negative feelings, embarrassment, anxiety, excessive strain, or a critical relative, on the other hand, can inhibit the let-down reflex and impair nursing. In fact, failure of the let-down reflex is, according to Karen Pryor in *Nursing Your Baby*, "the basic cause of almost every breastfeeding failure."[2]

Some hospital nurseries routinely give a bottle of sugar water to quiet the baby. Avoid this by rooming-in or by giving specific instructions to the staff. The bottle interrupts the supply-and-demand process of milk production. In addition, the baby may get used to the rubber nipple and have a harder time taking milk from the breasts.

By giving birth in a peaceful environment surrounded by supportive persons, you are already taking a giant step toward successful nursing. If you plan a hospital birth, rooming-in is most conducive to nursing your baby. The baby's immediate physical presence will help you fulfill his needs quickly and efficiently. Later, at home, a supportive partner (as well as the absence of unsupportive friends and relatives!) will aid nursing immensely.

Benefits of Nursing

The American Academy of Pediatrics recommends breast milk as the infant's primary source of nutrition for the first six months of life.

Breast is best, as the saying goes, for a number of reasons that will benefit you, your partner, and your baby.

• The baby will be healthier. Specifically designed for human babies, breast milk is more easily digestible than cow's milk. Your milk and the colostrum that precedes it contain antibodies and immunologic factors to protect your baby from various diseases. The bacteria in the breastfed baby's intestinal tract is considerably different from that in the bottle-fed baby's intestines. The nursed baby is less likely to develop intestinal viruses.

• Nursing is the most natural way to feed a baby.

• No baby is allergic to mother's milk, although the baby may be allergic to something in the mother's diet that may be transferred through the milk. This is easily corrected by altering your diet.

• Nursing affords total mobility. The baby can be fed any time, any place, with no preparation. Breast milk is always available and at the perfect temperature. There are no 2 A.M. bottles.

• Nursing is less expensive than bottle-feeding.

• Nursing saves time on preparing formula and cleaning and sterilizing bottles.

- Nursing promotes healthy tooth and jaw development.
- The breastfed baby's stools are different and remarkably less odorous then the bottle-fed baby's.
- Nursing is the best way to fill the baby's emotional needs, provided the mother feels comfortable about nursing.
- Nursing is pleasurable to the mother.

Some new mothers feel that nursing will inhibit their freedom. Nursing does carry certain naturally built-in obligations. Either the baby has to be breastfed, or if mother and baby are separated, as is the case with working mothers, milk must be periodically expressed from the breasts (to be either discarded or saved for the baby's feeding in mother's absence).

If the mother wants to feel free to be away from her baby, she can always express a little milk and leave it in a bottle for a baby-sitter or the father. This way, the mother has some time to herself, and the father gets to feed the baby. If she prefers, she can use an occasional bottle of formula. Some mothers successfully combine nursing and bottle-feeding.

Expressing and Storing Breast Milk

You can easily express milk to fill a bottle for a baby-sitter, for storage, or to bring to the hospital for a sick or premature baby. Either express it manually or use a hand or electric pump. Some childbirth and nursing-mothers groups will loan or rent electric pumps. They are also available for clients' use at most maternity centers.

Milk will keep in a clean container in the refrigerator

for twenty-four hours. If you wish to store the milk for a longer period, freeze it. The hospital will probably provide a sterile container if your baby is in special care.

Defrost milk in the refrigerator before use. Placing the container in boiling water to thaw it will curdle the milk.

MANUAL EXPRESSION

Express the milk into a clean container.

With clean hands, place your thumb and forefingers on the areola (the darkened area around the nipple). Begin with the thumb above the nipple and the forefingers below. Press your thumb and forefingers together, compressing the breast while pushing back toward your chest.

Continue this at several places around the areola.

(Warm compresses applied to the breasts before manual expression will encourage the let-down of milk.)

An excellent source of information regarding breastfeeding is La Leche League's publication, *The Womanly Art of Breastfeeding*.[3]

Preparing for Breastfeeding during Pregnancy

For as long as mothers have been giving birth, women have been nursing successfully. Most have done nothing to prepare the breasts, beyond the common-sense basic of eating a healthy, well-balanced diet.

It is not necessary to do anything to prepare for nursing if you don't want to. Today, however, most American women's breasts are overprotected by bras and are rarely exposed to the sun. Though none of the following steps are essential to successful nursing, they may help to reduce nipple pain and contribute to a smoother start in breastfeeding your baby.

Though these steps are widely recommended by childbirth educators and in a variety of good books, some nursing experts believe they are ineffectual in reducing tenderness. They feel that the main benefit of prenatal breastfeeding preparation is to make the woman more comfortable touching herself, if that is difficult for her. However, frequent rubs with a terry cloth towel will make *any* area of the body less tender.

- Rub the nipples with a terry cloth towel after taking a shower.
- Do nipple rolling once or twice daily. Supporting your breast with one hand, take the nipple between the thumb and forefinger of the other hand. Pull it out firmly but not hard enough to cause discomfort. Roll the nipple between the fingers for one-half to two minutes.
- If you both agree, your partner can stimulate the nipples manually or orally.
- Expose the breasts to sun and air frequently.
- Avoid alcohol or alcohol preparations on the nipple or areola, as these dry the skin and may cause cracked nipples.

Many recommend breast massage and manual expression of a few drops of colostrum. But according to Marvin Eiger and Sally Olds in *The Complete Book of Breastfeeding*, these have not proven beneficial.[4]

Psychological and emotional preparation for nursing is as important, if not more important, than physical preparation. This is really something both partners must do. It is ideal if the mother is able to embrace nursing as a natural function and the best way to care for her baby. Meanwhile, the father should be able to see the breasts as other than sexual objects and be willing to "share the breast" with his child.

Few things in art or nature are more beautiful than the nursing mother. Though it is becoming increasingly common to see mothers nursing their babies in parks and other public places, many still feel that it is more acceptable to give a baby a bottle in public than to nurse. This sort of attitude is not without its effects on new mothers. Influenced by those around them, many are inhibited or have negative feelings—conscious or unconscious—about nursing. Until they have given birth themselves, many new mothers have never even seen a mother nursing!

Reading a good book about nursing (see Resources section at the end of this book), attending childbirth classes that are wholly supportive of nursing, choosing a caregiver who supports breastfeeding, and talking to other mothers who have nursed, will all help develop a positive attitude and appreciation for breastfeeding.

Making the Nursing Decision Together

In the 1920s, nearly 90 percent of mothers breastfed their babies. By 1948, with the popularization of formula and the illusion that it was "healthier" to bottle-feed, the figure dropped precipitously to 38 percent. Later, in 1970, the percentage of nursing mothers sank to the all-time low of 25 percent. Today, nursing has been "rediscovered" and the figure has soared to about 60 percent and is still climbing.

Virtually every woman who can conceive and give birth to a child can nurse her baby. Inability to nurse or genuine contraindications to breastfeeding are very rare, but include having had extensive breast surgery or having a disease such as hepatitis, which affects the milk. In addition, some couples choose to bottle-feed if either partner has strong negative feelings about nursing.

Of greater importance than how the baby is fed— breast or bottle—is the way you feel. The way you hold your baby and the love you share mean more to his overall health and development than any number of ounces of fluid he ingests. It is better to bottle-feed and enjoy it than to breastfeed with resentment.

If you are healthy, yet undecided whether to nurse or bottle-feed, it is preferable to begin nursing. Then, if you want to change your mind later, you can. But if you begin bottle-feeding and then change your mind, nursing is more difficult (but by no means impossible). Few who give nursing a chance will regret it. As Marvin Eiger and Sally Olds point out in *The Complete Book of Breastfeeding*, "This priceless chance to nurse your baby comes only once in each baby's lifetime. Make the most of it. You may count those nursing days among the most beautiful and fulfilling of your entire life."[5]

A couple conceives a child together and, it is hoped, raises that child together. Ideally, how the baby is fed should also be a joint decision. Nursing can be truly satisfying and successful only if both parents agree.

"My husband was the one who encouraged me to breastfeed," says Drusilla, who has been a La Leche League leader counseling nursing mothers for the last eight years. "He was breastfed and I wasn't. When the baby was born, someone gave me a copy of *The Womanly Art of Breastfeeding*. After reading it I began attending La Leche League meetings. I became more and more involved and became a leader myself."

Since nursing is an emotionally sensitive process, the father's support is an essential factor in success, while a negative attitude on his part can doom nursing to failure.

Many fathers who are initially opposed to nursing change their mind once they learn more about the subject. If your partner is reluctant about nursing, you might encourage him to speak with other fathers whose partners have nursed successfully, discuss your feelings with each other, and perhaps read books about breastfeeding together. The La Leche League publishes an excellent brochure on the father's role, "Father to Father—On Breastfeeding," by David Stewart.

Some fathers are not enthusiastic supporters of nursing because they suspect nursing will lower their partner's sexual desire (as some books suggest). Few fathers can be expected to support a process that will rob them of their own sexual fulfillment. But this is not the case with nursing. Nursing *never* contraindicates lovemaking. Breastfeeding and sexual desire are further discussed in Chapter 5.

Another reason some fathers are unsupportive of breastfeeding is that they feel isolated, left out. During a postpartum get-together of couples who had recently given birth, Myra said, "I chose to bottle-feed because I wanted my husband Bill to feel more involved and so he would be able to feed the baby whenever he wanted."

But the father *can* feel involved in the nursing process. He can even feed the baby now and then. For instance, the mother can express breast milk into a bottle. The parents can also supplement breastfeeding with an occasional bottle of formula. Though frequent formula-feeding may lead to nursing problems, a bottle now and then can give the mother a sense of freedom while offering the father greater participation.

The isolation some fathers feel regarding nursing is heightened by a number of unfortunate attitudes and customs.

"When we were considering nursing our expected baby," says Pamela, recalling her first pregnancy, "we contacted a local nursing-mothers' group to get information. A woman came to our home the next day. I was touched by her generosity until she later invited me to a meeting. When I asked my husband, John, who was sitting next to me on the couch, if he would like to go, the woman interrupted. She said that husbands could not come to meetings dealing directly with nursing, but were permitted only at general meetings. Needless to say, neither of us attended their meeting."

Unfortunately, this is not an uncommon story. In one childbirth class I visited, the men and women were separated into two groups during a discussion of breastfeeding. The men wondered what the women were doing, and the women talked about what the men were thinking.

Nursing advocates often refer to the mother and baby as "the nursing couple," which, though a beautiful phrase, says little for the father. It goes without saying that it is the woman who nurses the child. It is her body that manufactures the milk. Nursing is exclusively a female's function. But that doesn't mean that the father must be made to feel isolated or that he should be excluded by thoughtless customs. We now recognize the value of the father's presence during prenatal exams and the birth (as well as his right to attend). But we still have some distance to go when it comes to the subject of nursing.

One way to insure that the father is involved and supportive of nursing is to approach the subject as a couple. Explore nursing together. If you attend meetings for nursing parents, try to attend them together. Though the father cannot produce milk, he can be involved in nursing decisions, and he can share the act of nurturing his child.

WARNING SIGNS

Excessive bleeding and fever indicating infection are the major problems to watch for. If you develop either of these problems or any of the other signs listed below, consult your caregiver without delay.

* *Heavy bleeding is defined as soaking a large-size pad in less than two hours, or the persistent passage of golf ball–size clots.*

* *Fever after the first twenty-four hours indicates infection.*

* *Foul-smelling lochia indicates infection.*

* *Burning sensation during urination, or unusually frequent urges to urinate (especially when little fluid is passed) may indicate urinary tract infection.*

* *Soreness and redness in legs may indicate phlebitis, inflammation of the veins.*

* *Soreness or redness in breast(s) may indicate mastitis, inflammation of the breast.*

* *Feelings of depression, great anxiety, or inability to cope may indicate the need for counseling.*

THE SIX-WEEK CHECKUP

Four to six weeks after birth, your caregiver will examine you to make sure your body is returning to its nonpregnant condition without problems. Scheduling exams four weeks after birth is increasingly common.

The postpartum exam includes:

- Measuring your weight and blood pressure.
- A pelvic exam to see that an episiotomy or tears to the perineum are healing properly, to check the cervix, and to assess the size and position of the uterus to make sure uterine involution is complete.
- A breast exam to assess the condition of the breasts and nipples.
- A blood test to measure the iron content.

At this time, any possible problems can be treated, referrals made if necessary, and contraception discussed.

Don't hesitate to call your caregiver before your scheduled appointment should you have any problems or concerns.

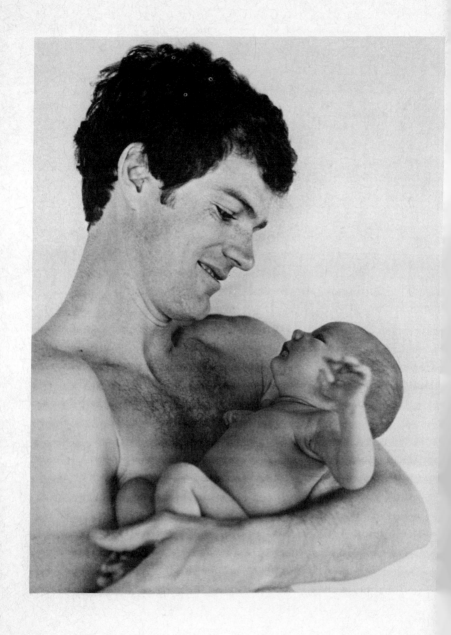

chapter three
· · · · · · · ·

Your changing emotions

The climax of pregnancy, birth is the most significant social and biological transformation in the lives of most couples. The birth of a baby is the beginning of a family. Labor is a rite of passage—in the figurative as well as the literal sense of the term. As the baby makes his passage to the world of extrauterine life, a couple becomes a mother and father, an older child becomes a brother or sister.

After the baby comes, your lives are quite transformed. Suddenly the overwhelming responsibility, sometimes joyful, sometimes frightening, of being a mother or a father dawns. You are now parents twenty-four hours a day, seven days a week, responsible for another human being who is wholly and utterly dependent on you. You must attend to the baby's almost ceaseless needs—to be fed, changed, kept warm and safe, played with, held, and loved.

You and your partner revolve around a new axis: your child. Your schedule is not the same. When the baby comes you are no longer master of your own time. Whatever you do, every time you wish to go out, even if only for a brief walk, there is the baby to consider.

Moreover, being a mother and father is forever. You can't turn back. For many this realization is utterly overwhelming. "I love my daughter intensely," says Sharon, the mother of a six-month-old baby. "But it took me a long time to admit that three days after she was born, there were times I didn't want her. Baby care was actually easier than I expected. But the thought of the responsibility was almost unbearable—she was really going to be my daughter the rest of my life!"

The responsibility of new parenthood can at times be enervating, especially when you are up in the middle of the night with a crying baby. Sometimes you may wonder how you can cope. And at other times parenthood can be the most wonderful thing that's ever happen to you.

For first-time parents especially, confronting their new roles may unleash a flood of conflicting emotions. The elation that so often crowns giving birth may be followed by doubts, insecurity, and feelings of inadequacy. In addition, many new parents feel trapped and robbed of their prepregnancy freedom. They may fear that their relationship with one another will never be as good as it was pre-baby. They may occasionally resent the baby, and then feel guilty for having felt this way. The "baby blues," discussed later in this chapter, can worsen such feelings.

After the birth of his first child, Anton said, "I was overwhelmingly excited in the hospital! Two days later when we brought the baby home and he was up crying half the night, I realized, here the baby was planted on us and we didn't know what to do with him!"

After her daughter, Courtney, was born, Cara recalls, "I was scared to death because I was supposed to know what to do but didn't. I also felt very frustrated the first few days. I loved Courtney. But I was so drained and she needed me so much. I wanted my husband, Kingsley—I felt so much closer to him all of a sudden and felt resentful that I couldn't just get the baby to sleep and be with him for a while. I was so used to spending time just with him. Now Courtney was with us twenty-four hours a day. On top of all this, I felt guilty for feeling the way I did."

Most couples make preparations for the new baby during pregnancy. They may buy clothes, diapers, a bassinet or cradle, rattles, mobiles, and so on. They prepare to make the baby happy in its new environment. But preparing themselves emotionally for the new role they will share is also important.

Discussing your feelings, both positive and negative, and your expectations about parenthood with your partner early in pregnancy will help you prepare for and assume your new roles with less stress. Whether or not you have confronted your feelings during pregnancy, however, you should certainly discuss them during the postpartum weeks.

It is also wise to talk to your partner or a friend about your feelings regarding your birth experience. Some women feel cheated or that they have somehow failed if things didn't go as they planned of if they had unwanted intervention. This is especially true of mothers who have given birth in hospitals. A frustrating birth experience can color the first few postpartum days or even weeks. But sharing your feelings will help.

It is normal to feel awkward, especially during the first few days, when you both will probably be very tired. New, inexperienced parents often doubt their ability to care for and nurture their child in the best possible way, to be a good mother, a good father.

During the early days, the inexperienced mother may be particularly vulnerable. Affected by a multiplicity of factors, both physiological and psychological, she will probably be sensitive to comments and criticisms from relatives, friends, and health professionals. Even well-intended remarks like the so-often-heard "Are you sure the baby's getting enough milk?" can be deflating. "Just when I would feel I was getting the hang of it, they would make me feel I had it all wrong," one woman said, recalling the first days of motherhood at home with her relatives.

The way birth has been viewed in this society affects a new mother's self-image, as well as the way she thinks about childbirth during pregnancy. In this country, birth has been approached almost as if it were an illness. Until just recently, pregnant women were treated like invalids in the majority of hospitals—confined to bed during labor, given routine intravenous feeding, hampered with restrictive policies about guests, and so forth. In a few hospitals women are still treated this way! The overall effect of such an approach to childbearing may leave the new mother feeling more awkward, more isolated, and less sure of herself than she might otherwise.

The new mother needs to be reassured, encouraged, praised, loved. Her partner is the best person to fill this need. But other sensitive and understanding family members, particularly her own mother, can be especially helpful in giving emotional support as well as practical advice—diapering, bathing, meeting the baby's needs. Parenting behavior is both instinctual and learned. The new mother needs to be reminded to trust both her maternal intuition and her ability to learn what she doesn't already know.

Your lives have acquired a new dimension. You and your partner have crossed a bridge to entirely different roles in life. It is awesome to realize that you have actually made what one author refers to as "a quantum leap into another generation."[1]

New motherhood can be especially difficult for the active career woman. Suddenly she finds herself at home with endless time alone with her baby. Being at home with an infant may make her feel especially dependent on her partner. She may feel ambivalent about staying at home, feel "unproductive," as if she is "not out in the real world" any more.

On the other hand, making the decision to continue working often causes ambivalence about motherhood. Should I be spending more time with the baby? Am I doing the right thing? Added to this is the expense of day care.

In a few cases, the father stays home while the mother works. He assumes the major part of the mothering role, which may be particularly difficult for him. However, greater difficulty adjusting often occurs when both parents are career-oriented.

No matter what the circumstances, having a baby adds a new perspective to a couple's relationship. It would be a mistake to paint a dark picture of new parenthood in an attempt to discuss coming to terms with the realities of the postpartum period, although responsibilities, frustrations, and fears are real. But there are also new discoveries and new joys, which new parents have never dreamed of before.

"The adjustment was difficult the first two days," Delores recalls, "but infinitely rewarding. When Reed was two weeks old we were already discussing having another child."

You will discover new pleasures—shared secrets and joys—that mean nothing to your friends who have no children. A certain facial expression, perhaps a sound, a particular habit your baby has that has special meaning only to the two of you. Then there are the tremendous moments that follow as the baby grows, unforgettable events to look forward to and to look back on later. Your baby's first step or his first gurgly word. Such simple things that we perhaps take for granted can unlock a reservoir of emotion.

Like the wind, the new parents' fluctuating emotions come and go—as if of their own inner accord. The best thing is to flow with the changes and move through them as your new family unfolds.

THE BABY BLUES

According to anthropologist Ashley Montague,[2] 80 percent of mothers who give birth in American hospitals suffer from that constellation of tears, irritability, and depression known as postpartum or *baby blues* (sometimes called *after-baby blues*). Ranging in intensity from a vague "down" feeling to inexplicable depression and frequent crying, postpartum blues occurs about the third to fifth day after birth and may continue for a period of a day or two to several weeks.

Leora, a new mother, experienced a period of postpartum depression that lasted a month and a half after her daughter was born. "I felt like everybody was against me—my husband, my mother, my sisters—everybody! Later I realized it was just my emotions."

Another mother said she was sad much of the time during the first few postpartum weeks. "The only thing that made me happy was my baby."

On the other hand, many mothers feel distressed on account of their baby! They feel the sudden pressure of the inescapable burden of having to care for a child.

Fathers, too, may experience baby blues. Your partner may need you as much as you need him.

The baby blues is so common and affects such a large percentage of new mothers that many childbirth professionals consider it a normal part of having a baby. But it is not inevitable. You can take several steps both during pregnancy and after the baby is born to reduce the intensity of, if not eliminate, postpartum blues.

A variety of factors both physical and emotional lend a hand in bringing on the baby blues. Mainly, it is a result of the way birth is approached in today's society. Without doubt, unnatural childbearing customs associated with hospital birth in this country are largely responsible for unpleasant postpartum, as well as disappointing birth experiences. The sterile, impersonal atmosphere, the overuse of pain-relief medication and hormonal preparations, the use of the central nursery, restrictive visiting policies, and the isolation of a mother from her family all affect the new mother's feelings. Happily such customs are changing and hospitals are becoming more comfortable places to experience a normal birth and follow-up. But caution in choosing a hospital is still essential.

A recent British study shows that depression occurs in about 60 percent of hospital deliveries, as compared to only 16 percent of home births.[3] This clearly indicates that the birth environment has a profound impact on a woman's experience of new motherhood.

The reason the incidence of postpartum blues is so much lower among home-birth than hospital mothers is presumably that at home babies and mothers are not usually separated. Generally speaking, at home there are minimal interruptions to the natural process. There are usually fewer stresses at home. You are on your own turf and more in control. This doesn't mean that you have to give birth at home to avoid the baby blues. Whether you birth at home, in a childbearing center, or in a hospital, you can create the atmosphere conducive to early parent-infant contact. If you choose your birth environment carefully and plan ahead, you can make the most of your first hours together and begin new parenthood as smoothly as possible.

There is no single overall cause of baby blues applicable to all new mothers. But contributing factors may include the following:

Maternal-infant separation during the first few hours after birth. "Postpartum blues are largely a psychological phenomenon of the woman who is separated from her family and her baby," writes Helen Varney, of the Maternal-Newborn Program at Yale University's School of Nursing, in her text *Nurse-Midwifery.*[4] Removal of the newborn from his mother immediately or shortly after birth is probably the most significant causative factor of postpartum depression, creating emotional anguish and trauma for both mother and child.

The first hour after birth, as previously discussed, is an emotionally sensitive time for mother and baby. Separation from family and prolonged hospital stay can increase the severity of depression after birth and interfere with adaptation to motherhood.

To avoid emotional trauma caused by maternal-infant separation, simply remain with your newborn. Unless there are complications, you, your partner, and baby can stay together right on the bed where you have given birth. Even if there are medical complications, you can still remain together, as discussed in Chapter 1.

Confronting your new and irreversible roles as mother and father. During pregnancy, the focus is often on preparing for a safe, happy birth. Though most parents-to-be make preparations at home for the baby, many don't take the time to reflect on what it will be like to have a new family member.

Then the baby is born and everything changes precipitously, dramatically, and permanently. Suddenly you discover that you are a mother, your partner a father.

You can't avoid the flood of emotions that will inevitably follow birth. In fact, trying to push them aside or refusing to express them may lead to more serious problems and even prolonged depression.

Under most circumstances, however, you can avoid situations that tend to intensify negative postpartum feelings, such as maternal-infant separation, prolonged hospital stay, and inadequate preparations at home.

Discussing your negative as well as positive feelings with your partner; having realistic expectations of one another; the father taking vitally important paternity leave to be with his family; and making advance arrangements for help at home, are all-important steps that will make confronting your new and irreversible roles much less traumatic.

Sorrow that pregnancy is over and the baby no longer in the womb. Throughout pregnancy, the expectant mother experiences a sense of unity with her unborn child. After the fourth prenatal month she can feel it moving, turning, kicking, and hiccupping. This sense of physical oneness with the baby abruptly ends with birth.

Andrea, the mother of a baby girl, said, "I felt empty those first few days. I could hardly believe the baby was no longer part of me." Many new mothers feel empty and suffer a period of minor grief after birth, when the living presence of their baby is no longer within their body.

After her child was born, Greta recalls: "I had very much enjoyed the feeling of being pregnant and the fullness. When you're walking down the street, everyone knows how special you are. When the baby was born, I felt an emptiness inside—especially when I wasn't right with the baby."

Though common, this reaction is by no means universal. When she read about feeling loss over the fact that the baby was no longer inside, my wife, Jan, said, "It seems strange. How could I possibly grieve that the baby is not inside when I have him to hold in my arms?" Jan did, however, miss pregnancy somewhat because she found the prenatal months among the most enjoyable in her life.

Under normal circumstances, the feeling of loss is usually mild and no cause for baby blues, though it may be a contributing factor. However, the sense of loss can be exacerbated by maternal-infant separation, and then it becomes a pertinent issue.

Prolonged skin-to-skin and eye-to-eye contact immediately after birth, and nursing the baby on demand, will mitigate any feelings of sorrow that the baby is no longer part of one's body.

Loss of "center of attention" status. "It seemed no one cared about me any more," said Martha, recalling the early days after the birth of her first child. "All they asked about was the baby." Such is the experience of the majority of new mothers.

Pregnant women tend to be the center of attention. Relatives and friends ask how you feel, what your plans are. They take a special interest in your changing body. Even strangers seem to care, helping with groceries, beginning conversations in the store or on the street, offering a seat on the bus. It is as if you are surrounded by an aura of good will.

Then suddenly, at the moment of birth, the attention is abruptly transferred to the newcomer. The mother's role is shifted from receiving care to taking care of another.

"Mothering the mother" is the best remedy. This is discussed later in this chapter. You need and deserve attention during this stressful phase of your life, perhaps more so than during pregnancy. Your partner's arranging for paternity leave, and the help of family and friends around the home will go a long way toward fulfilling *your* needs as well as the baby's.

Hormonal changes. Hormonal changes that accompany the onset of lactation and the return of the reproductive organs to their nonpregnant condition are thought to be one of the causes of the new mother's fluctuating emotions. There is little you can do about your changing hormones. But you can cooperate with the natural rhythm of your body—and thereby help create the conditions for a smooth after-birth recovery—by breastfeeding immediately after birth, nursing on demand, and resting as much as possible.

Fatigue. Exhaustion after birth can magnify irritability and depression, or any of the negative feelings that might accompany your first few weeks of motherhood. Over an extended period fatigue, with or without other contributing factors, is enough to make anyone feel blue.

Physical discomforts. The common physical problems many new mothers experience during the early postpartum period—perineal pain as a result of an episiotomy, tearing, stretching or bruising during birth, breast engorgement, afterpains—contribute to blue feelings during the first few weeks of motherhood, and may certainly intensify depression. Fortunately, most of the common postpartum discomforts can be reduced by following the simple steps in Chapter 4.

Anemia and low energy following postpartum hemorrhage, and disappointment and fatigue following a difficult or complicated birth, also contribute to baby blues. Pay special attention to nutrition, get extra rest, get help around the house, and so on. If you have had a disappointing birth experience, discuss your feelings with your partner, a friend, or a supportive childbirth professional.

If depression builds to the point that you feel you cannot cope, or if you find yourself neglecting your own and your baby's care, you should seek professional counseling. Ask your caregiver for a referral. Also, see the list of resources at the end of this book.

Understanding the factors contributing to postpartum blues, and planning your birth and the time afterward carefully, will certainly help you enjoy a smoother postpartum recovery. But it will not guarantee that your first few weeks of motherhood will be free of tears, irritability, and frustration. Even if you and your partner do all in your power to make the transition to your new roles smooth, you may still experience the baby blues. This doesn't mean that you are an inadequate mother or in any way abnormal. It simply means that regardless of how well organized you are, how well you plan, even how much you love your child and want to be a parent, you cannot harness all the many unforeseen feelings that come with the new baby.

PATERNITY LEAVE

There is no time in a mother's life when she more needs her partner's assistance, support, and love than during the childbearing season. According to psychiatric social worker Lyn Delliquadri and psychologist Kati Breckenridge, writing in *The New Mother Care*, women whose husbands participate in birth experience fewer postbirth difficulties.[5] In most childbirth classes the emphasis is on the father's participation during labor. But the importance of the father's help after birth should not be overlooked.

In *Sharing Birth: A Father's Guide to Giving Support During Labor*,[6] I strongly urge fathers to be involved throughout the childbearing experience. Sharing his feelings with his partner during pregnancy, attending prenatal appointments together, and seeing birth as a family affair (rather than a clinical procedure) are the best ways to prepare for a safe, happy birth and to begin preparation for parenthood. In *Sharing Birth*, I also point out that emotional support and encouragement through labor not only reduce the fear and pain of labor, but in some cases even shorten labor's length and reduce the chance of complications, including the need for a cesarean section.

The father's role after birth is just as important. His presence and help in the hospital or childbearing center, and later, his presence at home, can strengthen the family bond, reduce the chance of his partner's experiencing postpartum depression, and make the sometimes rocky transition to new parenthood immeasurably smoother for both parents.

If birth takes place in a hospital or childbearing center, it is ideal for the father to remain with his partner *throughout* her postpartum stay (which need be only a few hours if she experiences a normal vaginal birth). He can talk with his partner and be with the baby, taking time out for the inevitable phone calls and visitors, of course.

Charlene, mother of an 8 lb. 6 oz. girl, spent the day of birth in the hospital birthing room where she had labored. "Melissa was born at 5:30 A.M. Afterward, Ray massaged me all over with coconut oil. Then we snuggled together with Melissa between us in the big double bed until late in the afternoon, when we went home. I couldn't help laughing when the pediatrician had to wake Ray up to do the newborn exam, just when he had gotten to sleep."

The father should plan to be home for about one week.

Though he may not be paid for the time he takes, the benefits of paternity leave far outweigh any financial loss. Besides, his first and primary responsibility during this highly sensitive time is to be with his partner and child as the new family develops.

Nothing will substitute for the father's presence. Though there may be other people to help out around the house and meet the new mother's practical needs, the father is still needed to cope with the emotional and spiritual realities of shared parenthood. His presence is the most effective way of sharing his love for his family.

Immediately after their daughter, Karen, was born, a breech vaginal birth, Leo took care of the baby while his wife, Susan, received intravenous medication for pre-eclampsia and had an episiotomy sewn. The following day the new family went home. "Leo stayed with me for a few days. It made a huge difference. I couldn't have gotten around without him!" Susan says.

David remained at home with his wife, Sharon, after their first child was born. "If the baby woke up and wasn't hungry, David would hold him, rock him, and change him. This gave me a chance to take much needed naps."

The father, as well as the mother, can assume baby care. After an initial period of skin-to-skin and eye contact, he can diaper and dress the baby, or perhaps just enjoy mutual exploration. As one new father involved with his partner in the care of their baby boy said, "I changed him; she nursed him; she rocked him; I burped him."

At home, there are innumerable ways he can help. He can cook, clean, and do the laundry, as well as share baby care. If there are other children, he should spend extra time with them—they will need special attention too!

Bill, the father of two girls, said, "We spent as much time with my six-and-a-half-year-old daughter as with the baby. She was extremely jealous at first and needed extra attention and affection."

The father's presence and attention, however, are more important than any specific tasks he performs. After the birth of his daughter, Caitlyn, Rob took a leave of absence to be home with his wife. Kim recalls: "I was forging a new identity, and knowing he was right there was really important. The most valuable thing he did was accept me as I was."

As mentioned before, a positive attitude on the father's part can spell the difference between breastfeeding problems and successful nursing. Of course, his taking paternity leave and being actively involved and supportive during the postpartum period will not guarantee that there will be no breastfeeding problems. But since nursing is most successful when the mother is calm, secure, and relaxed, his help will go a long way.

Often, special things are what count the most to the new mother. Bringing home dinner, even if it's just a pizza, or giving her a little gift, can mean a lot. Above all, the new mother wants to know that she's still attractive to her mate. Telling her "I care . . . I love you," is probably more important than anything else.

It goes without saying that the mother is the one who has experienced the physiology of labor. She has given birth. The father will probably be the stronger one afterward, able to help her through the recovery period. But he also may be tired at first—especially if he has given support through a long labor. Though my wife and I had both been up all night, after the baby was born she had far more energy than I had. All I had done was make dinner, sit on the bed with her through the night, giving labor support, and "catch" the baby when he was born, while Jan had labored and given birth to our son. Yet I was utterly exhausted from lack of sleep and excitement, not to mention the celebration wine at 6 A.M.!

The father, too, has needs. He needs to know that he is still loved, still desired. No one should expect him to forego his needs or think of himself as merely a support person for his partner. His life also is changing. He, too, has crossed the one-way bridge to parenthood.

Fathers often feel jealous when their partner's attention is caught up with the baby during the early days and weeks. No man wants to take second place to his child. Jealous feelings may be especially strong if the mother is nursing. The father may feel isolated, left out, perhaps even rejected. The fact that lovemaking may be precluded for a few weeks may heighten these feelings. (This is discussed further in Chapter 7.)

It is especially important to work together during this sensitive part of the childbearing season to fulfill one another's needs. After the first week, it helps to make time to be alone together, away from the baby. Go out to dinner or go for a walk, just the two of you.

The life-altering era after birth is a time to draw close to one another. Both parents need each other's attention, each other's reinforcement, and above all each other's love.

MAKING THE TRANSITION SMOOTHER

The physical and emotional transitions that follow birth are affected by everything from whether or not you've had an uncomplicated labor and birth to how much experience you've had with babies and how closely the reality of motherhood—the baby's physical appearance, sex, behavior, and so forth—fits your expectations. By preparing carefully with your partner, you can make the transition to new parenthood and the overall postpartum experience immeasurably smoother.

Here are some steps to take before the baby is born:

A Natural Follow-up

The more natural and normal the transition between labor and the first few days of new parenthood, the less likely that there will be severe emotional upset—either for you, your partner, or the rest of the family.

Unless there are medical complications, consider leaving the hospital shortly after birth (within twelve to twenty-four hours, or even sooner). At childbearing centers, new mothers almost always leave within twelve hours of birth. Yet hospitals and health-care providers have varying views about the appropriate postpartum stay. Some strongly urge remaining in the hospital for two or three days following vaginal birth; others feel comfortable with early discharge. If your hospital doesn't encourage early discharge, you can make special arrangements with your caregiver before birth.

On the other hand, some mothers prefer to remain in the hospital, not only for rest but to have the expert care of the staff. Cassandra, a mother of three, said, "With the first child I left the hospital a few hours after birth. Being at home wasn't so difficult. All I had to do was bring the baby to bed with me. But with the third child I decided to remain in the hospital for a couple of days of rest. I had more time alone with the baby than I might have had at home."

However, as mentioned earlier, under most circumstances home is usually the most restful and natural place to begin your family.

Returning to an empty house after sharing the birth can be a somewhat upsetting experience for the father. "There was a phone in the birthing room, and we spent quite a bit of time just calling friends and relatives and sharing the news," Anton recalls of the hours after the birth of his son. "But when I finally went home, the house seemed very empty. I wanted to keep on sharing the news with people, but there wasn't anyone else to share it with. All the action was back in the hospital."

Remaining together—the new family—is the best natural follow-up to a shared birth. In many childbearing centers (and a very few hospitals) the entire family, including children, can remain in the same room or suite until the mother goes home.

Help at Home
Limit your activities to taking care of yourself and your baby for the first week or longer. Consider making some meals before the baby is expected and putting them in the freezer to minimize cooking time later. Otherwise, perhaps your partner, a relative, or friend can take over the cooking for a while. Some couples have relatives and friends who take turns bringing meals. Or your partner may be able to bring home take-out food.

"Having a wonderfully relaxed situation at home

made all the difference in the world," Courtney recalls. "Friends rotated helping me with the housework and cooking."

Particularly if you have other children, get help from your partner, relatives, or friends. You'll probably find just taking care of yourself and your baby quite exhausting for the first week or so.

So often one hears the well-meant advice: "Let the cleaning go." However, few things are more depressing than being exhausted and having to look at a messy house. You'll probably spend most of your time indoors for the first few days, so you'll no doubt want your home looking its best. Besides, having just given birth, you deserve the best possible surroundings! "If the house had been disorganized," said Mary Ellen, a midwife with a baby boy, "it would have taken its toll on me emotionally. So I got the house together toward the end of pregnancy and made sure someone was around to help me afterward."

Your partner may be able to take care of the cleaning as well as the cooking. But this shouldn't take precedence over being with the family. The father, too, will want time to enjoy his new baby and get accustomed to his new role. After the birth of their second child, Hannah's husband, George, took a week off from work to help out at home. But he got carried away. Every minute of the day he was doing something: cooking, cleaning, fixing things. Hannah recalls: "Finally I cried, 'Never mind the house or what needs to be done. Just sit and talk with me. Don't leave me and the baby by ourselves all the time.' "

You and your partner may consider hiring a temporary housekeeper to come in for a few hours once or twice a week. A hired housekeeper is an excellent suggestion for a friend or relative looking for a birth gift.

Other family members can do much to make the first weeks after birth smoother and less stressful for the new parents. I'll never forget how much it meant to us when my own mother helped Jan and me after our second son, Paul, was born. She stayed with us for a few days, cooked, cleaned, shopped, and even took little trips with our two-year-old son Carl.

Don't refuse offers of help. This new and trying era is no time to be self-sufficient. It is quite appropriate to depend on your own family and perhaps friends for a few days or longer. "Erin and I gave birth at home," said Jana, the new mother of twins. "We had several guests both at the birth and in the never-to-be-forgotten weeks that followed. My mother brought us cooked food almost every day. My best friend brought desserts that, though I hardly needed extra calories after gaining sixty pounds during pregnancy, were immensely appreciated. There was always someone offering to clean house, do the laundry, or something. But of course when you have twins, everyone wants to help out—and see the babies."

Family members and friends should focus on the new parents' needs and helping out at home rather than assuming baby-care responsibilities. Of course, grandparents will find it irresistible to spend some time with baby care. Nor can anyone expect someone, however close, to do housework without being allowed to enjoy the best part! But baby care should be kept to a minimum. In general, the new parents should have this role and learn to trust their own ability.

Mary Ellen Doherty, a certified nurse-midwife at

Emerson Hospital in Concord, Massachusetts, offers valuable advice to new parents about relatives: "Talk to them ahead of time about helping. Tell them you want to take care of the baby, but you would like them to give you a break now and then with baby care *without taking over*. Meanwhile, the biggest help they can give is with housekeeping, making meals, doing laundry, and other things that free you to spend more time with the baby."

When her mother and other relatives visited after the birth of her first child, Kathy recalls, "They all wanted the baby to stay out in the kitchen with them while I went to sleep. But I couldn't sleep. I just wanted them to give me back my kid and stop telling me what to do." When her next child was born, Kathy decided to outline clearly the role of others visiting her house. "They can sweep the floor, cook, do anything they want. But when it comes to the baby, they're limited to holding her now and then."

Too many visitors, even visitors who are helping out, can be exhausting for the new parents. You and your partner will have to decide on a happy balance for yourselves.

Some couples prefer to be by themselves as much as possible until they are more used to their new parenting roles. As one father said, "For the first two weeks we pretty much put other people off so we could be together—just the three of us."

The Professional Postpartum Helper
Anyone, male or female, can help a woman and her partner through labor and through the postpartum period following.

In many areas there are persons—usually childbirth

educators, nurses, midwives in training, or women who have given birth—who help childbearing women on a professional basis. Some give both labor support and assistance after the baby is born. Others focus exclusively on one or the other.

The services of a professional postpartum helper, sometimes called a *doula* (an unfortunate name meaning "slave") may include everything from house cleaning to suggestions on breastfeeding. Many take vital signs (temperature, pulse, and respiration) and examine the mother to insure her recovery is progressing smoothly. The experienced postpartum helper is also able to appreciate the new mother's emotional changes and offer much practical advice.

New parents who do not have family members living nearby may find the services of a professional postpartum helper particularly beneficial.

Resources
Be sure to have plenty of practical resources at your fingertips. These should include the telephone numbers of your caregiver, pediatrician, childbirth educator, relatives and friends, someone to help at home, baby-sitter, La Leche League or other nursing-mothers' group. See the list of resources at the end of this book for ideas.

Mothering the Mother
During the first day or so after birth, the new mother will probably be especially dependent on others for help. Not only is she apt to be tired, but she probably still feels vulnerable and in need of care as well. At the same time, it is important that she and her partner have the primary responsibility for baby care—not a nurse, a rel-

ative, or a friend. Essentially, the new mother is in a position for caring for another and being cared for at the same time.

We tend to overlook the mother's needs after the baby comes when attention is quickly diverted to the new arrival. Gifts, for example, are almost invariably for the baby. Rarely is anything given to the new mother or new father whose lives have changed so dramatically.

Today, we are especially cut off from the new mother's needs as a result of the increasing emphasis on hospital birth, where women are in the hands of medical professionals. Without devaluing the benefits of medical help, we can nevertheless generalize that for most women what is needed more is the presence of her partner, her family. As more couples are becoming conscious of the emotional benefits of out-of-hospital birth or early discharge, the needs of new mothers are once again coming into relief.

Traditionally, the mother's own mother and other female relatives who have given birth visit the house and cater to the new mother's needs. (This does not mean that the grandfather and other men in the family cannot be involved as well.) The benefit of their experience helps the woman get started in her new role and eventually branch off and find her own way of being a parent.

But the most important figure in meeting the new mother's needs is her partner. He should remain with her for twenty-four to forty-eight hours after birth, at the very least. There are many things he can do besides housekeeping and sharing baby care: he can help her bathe, give her a massage with a scented oil, or just sit and talk with her.

Understandably, the new father probably wants to share the news with all his friends as soon as possible. This is something most men want to do when the wave of elation is at its peak. No father should feel guilty for taking the time to make phone calls or greet a few friends at the height of the excitement. But at the same time he should bear in mind that his first responsibility is to his partner, to be with her and share his love.

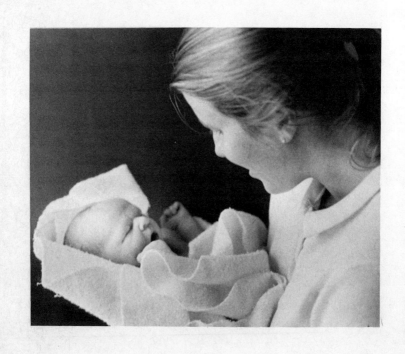

chapter four
. . . .

Relieving the minor postpartum discomforts

The minor discomforts that often accompany the first few weeks of motherhood may seem anything but minor to the woman overwhelmed with her new role. Discomfort can interfere with the mother's enjoyment of her baby, the baby care she provides, and her relationship with her partner. Physical problems—at a time when the new mother is so busy, yet so tired—can also exaggerate the blue feelings many new mothers feel.

Good nutrition, regular exercise, plenty of rest, and a natural birth are your best insurance for a healthy postpartum recovery. But no matter how well you prepare, nothing will guarantee that the weeks following birth will be discomfort-free. Even if you have no tears, hemorrhoids, and so forth, there are bound to be little complaints. As one new mother put it, "It was the little aches and pains that got to me: the bottom, the boobs, the head—all were hurting. The baby's constant crying gave me a headache that was made worse because I was frustrated that I couldn't just jump right up and go get him every time he cried."

Though the common problems discussed in this chapter are considered normal, fortunately you don't have to sit back and suffer with them. Some of the discomforts discussed ahead can be avoided by taking preventive steps during pregnancy. All can be reduced, if not entirely relieved, after birth.

Prevention is always preferable to cure. For those who are reading this book during pregnancy, preventive measures are included with the discussion of specific discomforts wherever appropriate.

A brief discussion of the cause of each discomfort and effective relief measures will be followed by warning signs of possible problems. If you experience any of these, consult your caregiver without delay.

AFTERPAINS

Afterpains, also called after-birth pains, are laborlike cramps resulting from the uterus alternately relaxing and contracting. Ranging from mild to severe, afterpains usually occur shortly after birth and disappear within a day or two, or at most a week. Afterpains may be more intense during nursing because the baby's sucking causes the flow of oxytocin, which intensifies uterine contractions. Relaxation and contraction of the uterus is also more pronounced following subsequent births, and afterpains may be more severe and continue for a longer time than in the first-time mother.

Relief measures consist of keeping the uterus contracted.

• Urinate frequently. A full bladder displaces the uterus and prevents it from remaining contracted. Emptying the bladder is sometimes enough to relieve afterpains.

• First be sure the bladder is empty; then lie in a prone position with a pillow under the lower abdomen. This puts pressure on the uterus, causing it to remain contracted. Cramps may intensify for a short while before relief is felt.

• Use an analgesia according to your caregiver's recommendation.

Warning: Extreme tenderness or severe, persistent cramps may be a sign of infection or an indication that the uterus is not involuting properly (see pages 23–28). Consult your caregiver without delay.

PERINEAL PAIN

The major postpartum complaint for new mothers, perineal pain ranges from soreness to acute discomfort. Perineal discomfort results from tearing during birth, having had an episiotomy, and stretching or bruising of the perineal tissues and muscles.

Discomfort from an episiotomy or large tear is usually greater than that resulting from a minor tear or the discomfort of a stretched and bruised, but intact, perineum. The tissues in the area swell and pull against the stitches, resulting in soreness. Swelling usually begins to subside by the third postpartum day. Soreness, however, may last a few weeks or longer.

The stitches used to repair an episiotomy or tear are rarely visible and are generally on the inside. They dissolve within ten days or at most two to three weeks. As this happens you may see flecks of threadlike material on a sanitary napkin. This is normal.

The key preventive factors in reducing (or eliminating) perineal pain are preventing tearing and avoiding an episiotomy.

Tearing

You were designed to stretch around your baby with a minimum of tearing, if any, and to return to your prepregnant shape in a relatively short time. Whether or not a tear occurs when the baby is born depends largely on four factors: the condition of the perineal tissue and musculature; your ability to relax and surrender to the labor process; the size and position of the baby; and the skill of your caregiver.

Your birthing environment will also influence your labor and the possibility of tearing. As British midwife Chloe Fisher points out, "A calm and unhurried atmosphere with a comfortable and confident woman can greatly affect the degree of relaxation and elasticity of the perineum."[1]

Large tears will probably be stitched. Minor nicks and tears will heal by themselves.

PREVENTING TEARING

You can greatly reduce your chance of tearing or minimize the extent of it by following several simple steps during pregnancy and labor:

• Exercise the pelvic floor regularly throughout pregnancy. See "The Blossom" exercise, pages 99–100.

• Do *perineal massage* during the final month or two of pregnancy and again before the head is born. Perineal massage increases awareness of the pelvic floor, increases circulation, and is said to promote stretching.

During pregnancy, you can do perineal massage yourself, or your partner can do it. During labor, your partner or your caregiver can do it for you.

Insert one or two fingers into the vagina and gently make half circles downward and toward the anus for two to three minutes. The increased vaginal secretions of pregnancy often provide adequate lubrication. Otherwise you can use a lubricant such as vitamin E oil or K-Y jelly.

Note: Check with your caregiver to be sure you don't have vaginitis, herpes, or other vaginal problems, as perineal massage may worsen or spread these conditions.

• Choose a supportive caregiver who is willing to help you give birth with an intact perineum.

• Choose a comfortable, peaceful birthing environment.

• Choose a comfortable birthing position and vary the position as you feel the need. Squatting or upright positions are usually most efficient for difficult births.

• Use warm compresses against your perineum during the bearing-down stage of labor. Your partner or caregiver can hold the compresses in place for you.

• Avoid bearing down forcefully when the baby's head is being born.

• Think of yourself as an opening flower. Keeping

this image in mind helps many mothers surrender to (rather than resist) the unfamiliar sensations of birth.

Episiotomy

A surgical incision made to enlarge the birth outlet as the baby is born, the episiotomy is by far the most significant cause of perineal pain. In most cases, it is also easily avoidable.

This procedure may be appropriate in unusual medical emergencies when the baby is severely distressed. However, some physicians and midwives *routinely* cut this incision, whether or not there are problems. The routine episiotomy is a custom peculiar to U.S. medical professionals and a subject of hot debate. Those in favor of the incision argue that it shortens the birth process and substitutes a neat, easier-to-repair cut for a jagged tear. Those opposed say the incision has no place in normal birth, is far larger than most natural tears, more painful during the postpartum period, and should be cut only in medical emergencies.

Though the episiotomy is not painful while being cut, the stitched incision can cause considerable postpartum discomfort.

It is important to realize that perineal pain resulting from an episiotomy is neither an inevitable nor normal part of childbearing. As the above-quoted British midwife, Chloe Fisher, states, "We should be making every effort to avoid it . . . There is no doubt that early feeding problems arise because the mother can't find a comfortable position."[2]

Since caregivers have different policies regarding this common surgical incision, it becomes the responsibility of the expectant mother to interview and choose her caregiver with this, among other things, in mind. To avoid episiotomy discomfort, look for a caregiver who is confident in your ability to birth naturally and who does an episiotomy only if there is a medical emergency (if at all).

RELIEVING PERINEAL PAIN

The following will help reduce swelling and ease discomfort from a tear, cut, stretching, or bruising.

• Apply ice wrapped in a washcloth to the sore area. (Don't apply the ice directly.) An effective remedy, ice numbs the perineum and also prevents or reduces swelling. Use ice packs for twelve to twenty-four hours after birth. Feel free to ask for ice if you are in a hospital where it hasn't been offered.

• After the first twenty-four hours, use warm water to soothe discomfort. In a hospital or birthing center, pour warm water over the perineum from front to back. This helps reduce the possibility of infection from anal bacteria. At home, take warm baths. Be sure someone is nearby if you feel dizzy or have difficulty getting out of the tub.

• Take warm sitz baths.* You might want to take an herbal sitz bath, ginger for itching, comfrey for healing.

• Place a heat lamp more than one foot from the perineum to promote healing. Use with caution and to avoid burning don't use if ointment has been applied.

• Apply witch hazel compresses to the sore area. Pour

---

* A sitz bath is a bath taken in a sitting position. Most hospitals have special tubs for this purpose. There are also portable sitz baths.

witch hazel over four-by-four gauze squares and ring out. Be sure your hands are very clean. Or, you can buy commercially prepared pads, like Tucks.

• In the hospital, numbing sprays and pain-relief medication are available.

• A compress of comfrey leaves helps facilitate healing. (Comfrey is available from many health-food stores and stores specializing in herbs.)

• If you find sitting uncomfortable, tightly draw up the pelvic floor (as if you were trying to hold back from urinating) before seating yourself, and hold the muscles until you are sitting. This avoids direct pressure on the stitched site. This is most helpful if yours is like most episiotomies, in which the incision goes directly from the back of the vagina toward the anus (midline episiotomy). If the incision angles off to one side (the less common mediolateral episiotomy), drawing up the pelvic floor sometimes heightens discomfort. Use cushions. It it helps, sit to one side so pressure is not directly on the sore area.

TO HASTEN HEALING

• Walk frequently. This stimulates circulation

• Eat a nutritious, well-balanced diet with plenty of protein and vitamins A and C to promote tissue growth and repair.

• Do pelvic-floor exercises to promote circulation and strengthen the pelvic-floor musculature (see "The Blossom," pages 99–100).

• Expose the area to air frequently.

Warning: Consult your caregiver if the pain or swelling is severe or worsens with time.

BREAST ENGORGEMENT

When the milk "comes in," the breasts sometimes become overfull, swollen, and tender. Engorgement, a condition in which the breasts become so full that the skin may be tight and shiny, results from pressure of increased milk, lymphs, and blood. Breast engorgement usually occurs about the second to fourth day after birth and lasts twenty-four to forty-eight hours.

TO PREVENT

- Begin breastfeeding immediately after birth.
- Nurse your baby on demand without *any* supplemental feedings for the first few days.
- Nurse from both breasts at each feeding, alternating the breast from which you begin feeding each time. This helps prevent milk from building up.

If the breasts become heavy and engorged despite preventive measures, try the following:

TO RELIEVE (NURSING MOTHER)

Relief measures consist basically in keeping the milk flowing and emptying the breasts.

- Apply a washcloth soaked in very warm water to encourage the milk to flow.
- Take a warm shower or bath to relieve discomfort and encourage milk flow.
- If the breasts are very full and taut, express a little milk before nursing so the baby can get a better grasp on the nipple. (See page 37)
- Massage breasts gently during feeding to improve milk flow.

- After nursing, express extra milk if the breasts still feel full and heavy.
- Use ice packs between feedings to reduce swelling and discomfort.
- Wear a supportive nursing bra.
- If necessary, take aspirin or acetaminophen to relieve pain and reduce mild fever.

TO RELIEVE (NON-NURSING MOTHER)
Do not remove milk in an attempt to relieve pressure. This stimulates further milk production and will prolong engorgement. Don't apply warm water or put any other heat source to the breast to soothe discomfort, as this encourages the milk to flow, which in turn will lead to more milk production.

- Use a supportive bra or bind a towel tightly around the breasts to ease discomfort. The breasts should be held up and in and be well supported.
- Use ice packs to numb the area.
- Take aspirin or acetaminophen to relieve pain and reduce mild fever.

Warning: Severe or persistent pain, warmth, redness, or hardness in the breasts may be signs of infection.

SORE OR CRACKED NIPPLES
Many women experience some nipple soreness, especially on the second or third postpartum day, when they

are first getting used to nursing. Women with fair skin, red hair, and those with sensitive skin are most likely to have sore nipples. The nipples may look red and chapped and may possibly even bleed. However, the problem is common and will usually heal by itself.

TO PREVENT

Toughening the nipples during pregnancy, using the steps outlined in Chapter 2, will often prevent sore nipples. Avoid alcohol and soap, which dry the nipples and may contribute to cracking and resultant soreness. The Glands of Montgomery (little bumps throughout the areolae) secrete a lubricating material that keeps the nipples protected.

If soreness does not go away on its own, try the following:

TO RELIEVE

- Dry nipples after feeding.
- Apply plain unmedicated lanolin or a mild cream such as Vitamin A and D ointment after each feeding. Wipe it off before nursing.
- Use absorbent bra linings and change them often.
- Expose nipples to air.
- Expose nipples to sunlight or a sunlamp (be careful of burning, especially if you use a lamp).
- Try manual expression before a feeding to get the milk flowing.
- Nurse from the less-sore breast first (unless they are equally sore). The baby often sucks hardest when beginning to nurse. By the time he is ready for the sore breast his nursing will be less vigorous.

- Change the baby's position often so that pressure will not always be on the same area of the breast.
- Use aspirin or acetaminophen before a feeding or ask your caregiver for an analgesia.
- If necessary, nurse for shorter periods of time (but frequently), giving the baby a pacifier to satisfy sucking needs.
- Sloane Crawford, C.N.M., in private practice in Brookline, Massachusetts, suggests applying a wet comfrey teabag to the nipple for fifteen to twenty minutes three to four times daily. Let air dry.
- Some midwives recommend using "Bag Balm." "This is more effective for relieving sore or cracked nipples than any other remedy," asserts Mary Ellen Doherty of Emerson Hospital in Concord, Massachusetts.

Bag Balm is an ointment manufactured for cows, packaged in an attractive container with a picture of a cow on the front and directions for applying the preparation to the udder! The balm should be washed off thoroughly before nursing. For further information, the label suggests, "Consult your veterinarian"! Bag Balm is available from the Dairy Association Co., Lyndonville, Vermont, 05851, and at local grain and feed stores.

Consult your caregiver if sore or cracked nipples persist or worsen despite relief measures.

FATIGUE
A period of high energy, elation, and excitement usually follows birth. But it is also normal to be exhausted after the baby is born, especially if you have had a long labor, were given medication, or other forms of medical intervention were used.

In any case, you are bound to experience some physical and mental exhaustion during the days and weeks that follow birth. The major causes of postpartum fatigue are: the physical exertion of labor; dramatic changes as the body begins to return to its nonpregnant condition; hormonal changes as lactation is established; taking care of the baby; changing emotions accompanying the sudden realization of a new, overwhelming, and irreversible role; and, of course, lack of sleep.

The best remedy is rest. But with a new baby this is not always possible. By sharing responsibility, both in the hospital and at home, the father can help you get much needed rest.

TO PREVENT EXCESSIVE FATIGUE
• Follow the steps for "Making the Transition Smoother" in Chapter 3, pages 64–71.
• Make advance arrangements for help around the house.

TO RELIEVE
• If you birth out of home, return home within twenty-four hours unless there are medical problems. Hospitals are generally not restful places.
• Limit the number of visitors.
• Try sleeping when the baby sleeps.
• Share the baby's care with your partner.
• Make arrangements to spend time by yourself or alone with your partner.

As already discussed, by taking paternity leave to care for you and the baby, your partner can significantly reduce your fatigue, though he also may need to rest—especially if he has been up with you through a long labor.

DIFFICULT OR PAINFUL URINATION

You may not feel the urge to urinate after birth, even when your bladder is full, as a result of pressure and stretching and the resultant desensitization of the pelvic-floor area. In addition, urinating may be difficult at first due to swelling of the tissues around the urethra. A full bladder, however, can increase *afterpains*, prevent the uterus from contracting efficiently, and lead to postpartum hemorrhage. In addition, retaining urine for a prolonged period after birth may contribute to urinary tract infection. Accordingly, if you are in a hospital and you haven't emptied your bladder within eight hours, catheterization (removal of urine from the bladder by means of a plastic tube inserted through the urethra) may be prescribed.

You can usually stimulate urination by one or more of the following steps:

• Breathe deeply and relax while attempting to urinate.
• Contract and relax the pelvic floor several times (to stimulate urethral response).
• Run the tap water near the toilet. Peculiar advice though it is, this has proved helpful to many new mothers.
• Oil of peppermint in the toilet water often aids urination. Sloane Crawford, C.N.M., in private practice in

Brookline, Massachusetts, has found this an effective remedy with her clients.

PAINFUL URINATION

Painful urination may result if the urine passes over a cut or tear in the perineum. Follow these steps to relieve the problem:

• Try urinating standing up in the shower with the water running over you.
• With a plastic squeeze bottle (usually supplied by the hospital) or a pitcher, spray or pour warm water over the perineum during and after urination.
• Drink plenty of water to dilute the urine and lessen discomfort.

Warning: Internal burning after urination or an intense, painful, and unusually frequent need to urinate (especially if you pass only a few drops each time) may be signs of a urinary tract infection. Consult your caregiver.

EXCESSIVE PERSPIRATION

Profuse perspiration is common, sometimes lasting for a few weeks, after the baby is born. This helps the body rid itself of the extra fluid retained during pregnancy. Sweating is often more profuse at night.

Though annoying, postpartum perspiration is something you have to put up with. It is unwise to restrict your fluid intake in an attempt to prevent sweating. Your body needs the fresh fluid.

To alleviate the condition, change clothes frequently

and take showers more often. You may also want to change the bed linens more often than you ordinarily do.

HEMORRHOIDS
Dilated, enlarged veins of the anus or rectum, postpartum hemorrhoids are caused by the pressure of the baby's weight through pregnancy. They may protrude from the anus or be inside. Hemorrhoids are most painful for the first two or three days after birth as a result of pressure and stretching. They eventually shrink.

TO RELIEVE
- Apply witch hazel compresses or over-the-counter preparations for relief.
- Use ice packs to numb the area and help the hemorrhoids recede.
- Replace hemorrhoids gently in the rectum after a bowel movement. If you wish, use a rubber finger cot available in the hospital or pharmacy.
- Take sitz baths in very warm or hot water.
- Keep the stool soft by increasing fluids and eating fibrous foods such as bran and whole grains.

CONSTIPATION
It is not essential to have a bowel movement in the first three days after birth, especially if you haven't eaten solid foods during labor. The digestive system slows down considerably during labor. The bowels are usually

emptied shortly before birth with prelabor diarrhea. If not, they are emptied during birth.

Relaxed bowels and lax abdominal muscles following birth contribute to the possibility of constipation. Exercising the abdomen during pregnancy is a preventive measure.

Hemorrhoids and/or a tender perineum may make the new mother reluctant to strain during elimination. Many new mothers have a fear of tearing out the stitches if they strain, but this will not happen.

TO RELIEVE
• Eat a diet high in whole grains, fresh vegetables, and fruits. Drink plenty of fluids to encourage the bowels. Try prune juice, a natural laxative.
• Walk daily and do regular exercise.

Note: Laxatives affect the milk. Use a stool softener instead or ask your caregiver for a recommendation.

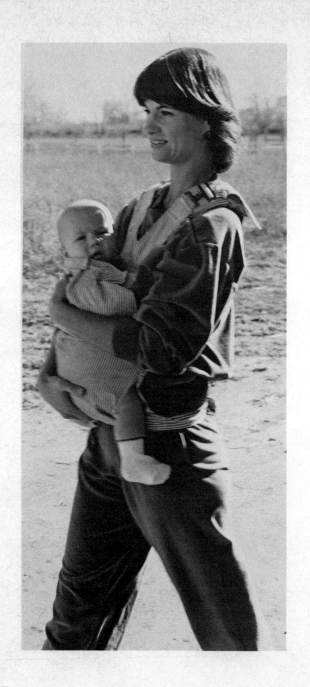

chapter five

Getting back in shape

Though childbirth will change your life irreversibly, it needn't permanently alter your figure.

The areas most stressed during pregnancy and childbirth are the pelvic floor, the abdominal muscles, and the back. These require the most attention after the baby is born.

The pelvic-floor musculature, which supports the uterus and its contents like a hammock, is considerably stressed. As mentioned before, a loose, saggy pelvic floor can result in decreased vaginal tone, urinary incontinence, and gynecological problems later in life. Exercising the pelvic floor is therefore of prime importance.

The abdominal muscles—depending on their prepregnant condition—may be weakened. Strengthening them is simply a matter of patience and regular exercise.

During pregnancy, the mother's center of gravity changes, predisposing her to walk with a somewhat arched back. Combined with lax abdominal muscles, this may contribute to backache, which may carry over after the baby is born.

Exercising regularly will restore the muscles and reduce your chance of being fatigued and uncomfortable during the postpartum period, helping you meet the demands of new motherhood.

One of the truly amazing things about the female body is its ability to create and nurture a child and then return to its prepregnant shape. But this doesn't happen overnight. Many new mothers expect to be slim immediately after the baby is born. But most discover that they cannot wear their favorite prepregnancy clothes right away. "I couldn't believe it!" recalls June after the birth of her daughter. "I couldn't button my old slacks around my floppy belly. I felt like I was still six months pregnant!"

The changes that accompany childbearing took nine months (actually ten 28-day lunar months). Fortunately, returning to your prepregnant shape will probably not take quite as long. It will, however, take several weeks and perhaps months after birth.

Average pregnancy weight gain is twenty-four pounds. This is only an average, and one should not attempt to hold the weight at this level. Lyn Jones, a nutrition educator and former executive director of the Midwifery Training Institute in Albuquerque, New Mexico, has found that most women she counsels gain thirty or more pounds. Some mothers gain more, some less. Quite a variation of normal weight gain is possible, depending on the individual.

My wife Jan gained ten pounds in her first pregnancy despite eating heartily. Since her prepregnant weight was only 102 pounds, we were both concerned that the baby wasn't developing properly (low birth weight is linked to a variety of complications). Yet the baby—healthy at birth—weighed seven pounds. During Jan's second pregnancy, her weight gain was similarly low, but by then we were able to accept this as normal for her body. We decided to abandon the scales during the third pregnancy! Other women with a similar diet have gained forty or more pounds.

Prenatal weight gain is not all baby. The baby, placenta, and amniotic fluid account for less than half of the additional weight. The remaining increase is the result of greater blood volume, retained fluids, retained fats, breast changes, fat deposits, and the increased size of the uterus.

Meanwhile, the abdominal muscles have been considerably stretched and will take some time to return to their former condition.

During the weeks that follow birth, the mother will lose much of this additional weight and her abdomen will eventually resume its former condition. However, the nursing mother probably will not lose all her pregnancy weight gain. She may retain an extra five to ten pounds in the form of fluids and fats. Assuming she is not overweight to begin with, she should accept the additional five to ten pounds as her normal weight as long as she is nursing.

Bear in mind that the somewhat floppy belly of the new mother is not really "out of shape" for this period in her changing life. Her temporary appearance is normal. There is quite a difference between the normal healthy changes that accompany childbearing—signs of the body's amazing creativity—and obesity.

The amount of weight gained during pregnancy will, of course, affect a mother's postpartum weight. However, upper limits on prenatal weight gain are not recommended. Eating a nutritious, well-balanced diet is essential for both the baby's well-being and a normal pregnancy and birth (and for successful nursing). But at the same time the mother should be aware that the weight gained in excess of twenty-four pounds may require additional effort to lose after birth.

Many women have neither the time nor the inclination to follow a regular exercise program. After all, the new mother undoubtedly has enough to do without adding a daily exercise routine to her already busy schedule! However, even if she doesn't wish to exercise regularly, every new mother should take the time to exercise the pelvic floor and tone the abdominal muscles, the former to help prevent gynecological problems and improve sexual response, and the latter to eliminate a floppy belly, help prevent backache, and allow her to be more comfortable in future pregnancies.

Getting in shape after birth will take less time if the mother is in good physical condition and has exercised throughout pregnancy.

EXERCISE GUIDELINES

Following are the basic guidelines for exercising safely and comfortably after the baby is born.

• Consult your caregiver before beginning an exercise program.

• Let your body be your guide. Tailor your postpartum exercises to your individual needs and preferences.

Some women detest the idea of a regular exercise program. They much prefer to get their exercise from outdoor activities. Aerobic exercises (those that benefit the circulatory and respiratory systems) are best for all-around conditioning. These include anything from walking, bicycling, and swimming to country dancing. Walking—especially if one can manage two to four miles a day—is the ideal exercise. Jogging may be hard on the lactating breasts and the back.

Hiking with the baby is excellent exercise as well as a wonderful way to calm a crying baby. Apparently the close quarters of the carrier, the motion, and the sound of your heart beating bring back memories of being in the womb.

Even if you are in good shape and choose to let outdoor activities fill your exercise needs, pay special attention to "The Blossom" and "Checking for Abdominal Muscle Separation" ahead.

• Ease into physical activity, particularly rigorous activity. Don't overexert. Fatigue or increase in the amount of lochia may indicate that you are doing too much too soon.

• Don't do any exercise to the point of pain.

• Stop exercising if you feel nauseated, dizzy, or faint.

• Avoid double-leg raises in the flat-on-the-back position and full sit-ups with both legs straight out during the postpartum period. These exercises can hurt the back.

During the early postpartum period, it is preferable to exercise twice or more in a day rather than to attempt multiple repetitions in one session.

Your baby can be with you while you work out, either

just watching or actually being involved in some of the exercises, making it a combination exercise and play period. Two books that recommend exercising with the baby and offer additional suggestions are: *Shape Up with Baby*, available from Pennypress, Seattle, Washington, and *Mommy and Me Exercises* by Christie Costanzo, available from Cougar Books, Sacramento, California.

You can begin the simpler exercises the first few days after birth. "Foot bending and circling," for example, (below) is only useful while you are still in bed, usually only the very first postpartum day. Others that you can do in bed either at home or in the hospital include "The Blossom" (pages 99–100) and "Abdominal Tightening" (page 101). Check the abdominal muscles for separation (pages 102–3) and if you find a gap, begin the "Chin-to-Chest" exercise (pages 103–4). You can also add "Pelvic Rocking in the Back-Lying Position" (pages 107–8). Wait until you feel up to it to add more.

Most of the exercises ahead are similar to those found in other postnatal exercise guides. (All tend to include many of the same, well-known, proven-to-be-beneficial exercises.) If you want additional exercises, see the resources section at the end of this book.

Note: The most important postpartum exercises are: "The Blossom," "Abdominal Tightening," "Checking for Separation of the Abdominal Muscles," and "Chin-to-Chest."

FOOT BENDING AND CIRCLING

Foot bending and circling is only of value while you are still in bed. At this time, bending and rotating the feet will help prevent blood clots by pumping the blood back from the lower extremities. If you are like many new mothers who are up and about the day the baby is born, you won't need these two exercises.

Foot Bending

1. Lie comfortably or semireclined, with back supported by pillows and legs elevated on a cushion or pillow.

2. Bend one foot back, toes as far toward the shin as possible.

3. Bend foot forward as far as you can.

4. Repeat 2–3 times.

5. Do the same with other foot.

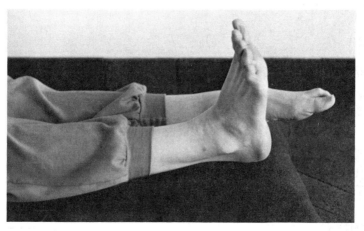

Foot bending

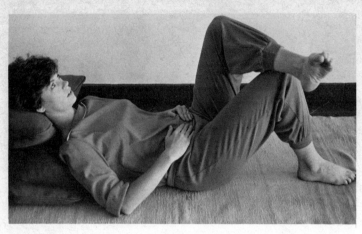

Foot circling

Foot Circling

1. Bend one leg at the knee and cross the other over the bent knee, leaving room to rotate the foot.

2. Make a circle with foot several times, first in one direction, then in the other.

3. Alternate feet and repeat.

4. You can also do foot circling in the same position as foot bending.

EXERCISING THE PELVIC FLOOR
Pelvic-floor tightening is the most important postpartum exercise.

No area of the body is more directly involved in the

birthing process than the pelvic region. As discussed earlier, the pelvic-floor musculature, called the pubo-coccygeus muscle, is considerably stretched and often left sagging after birth. Exercising the pelvic floor daily will tone the muscle, improve sexual response, and help prevent gynecological problems such as urinary incontinence and uterine prolapse (a condition in which the uterus slides down the birth canal).

Pelvic-floor tightening is sometimes called the "Kegel" exercise, after Arnold Kegel, a gynecologist who called attention to the importance of exercising the pubococcygeus.

The pubococcygeus muscle contracts when you try to stop the flow of urine. In fact, many childbirth educators suggest stopping and starting the flow of urine several times. This is a good way to get familiar with the action involved. Once you have a feeling for tightening the pelvic floor, try the following:

THE BLOSSOM

Introduced in *Sharing Birth: A Father's Guide to Giving Support During Labor,* this pelvic-floor exercise can be done in any position. At first you may be uncomfortable if you had stitches (but the stitches will not pull out). With practice, the exercise will become less uncomfortable.

You may feel as if you are getting nowhere with pelvic-floor exercises the first few days (or weeks) after birth. You may not feel the muscles in the vagina tightening at first. Don't be concerned. After all, the muscles and tissues have undergone tremendous stretching and perhaps bruising, especially if it was a difficult birth.

Keep up with the exercises, and be assured that this area will be restored.

1. Imagine that the inside of your birth canal is like a flower and that the flower is closing into a tiny bud, petal by petal, as you *gradually* tighten the pelvic floor.

2. *Draw up* the pelvic-floor muscles as tight as you can.

3. Hold for a few seconds.

4. Gradually release, feeling the flower blossom.

5. Repeat 5–20 times, several times daily. Increase the number of times if you wish.

As the pelvic-floor musculature gains strength, try doing this exercise in the squatting position, feet about shoulder width apart and flat on the floor, arms resting loosely on the knees.

THE POSTPARTUM ABDOMEN
After birth, the abdominal wall will probably be soft and flabby and the skin loose from having stretched during pregnancy. With exercise, good body mechanics, and good posture, the muscles will gradually regain their former size. Strengthening the abdominal muscles is particularly important as it will help you to regain your figure more rapidly, prevent backache, and keep the abdomen in condition for future pregnancies.

Avoid wearing a girdle. This holds in the abdomen but does nothing to strengthen or tone the muscles.

ABDOMINAL TIGHTENING

Holding in and tightening the abdominal muscles as you exhale is the simplest way to tone the belly. Do this in bed or in any comfortable position.

1. Breathe in deeply so that your belly rises as you inhale.

2. Now exhale slowly, pulling abdominal muscles as tight as you can, as if you were trying to make them touch your spine.

3. Hold for a few seconds.

4. Relax and repeat as often as you think of it throughout the day.

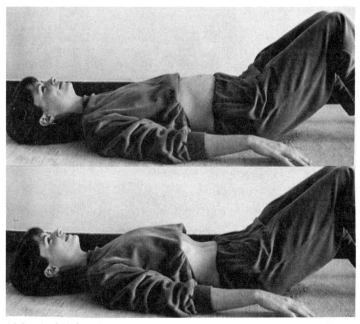

Abdominal tightening

CHECKING FOR SEPARATION
OF THE ABDOMINAL MUSCLES

As previously noted, the abdominal recti—a pair of muscles that run down either side of the abdomen in twin sheets—have a tendency to separate like a broken zipper during pregnancy. Known as diastasis recti, this separation is a common, painless condition, more pronounced in women who have borne children before. However, it can lead to both a flabby belly and back problems. The latter is particularly common during pregnancy, when the uterus sags forward against the weakened abdominal muscles and tugs on the spinal cord, to which it is attached by two ligaments.

You can check for separation of the abdominal muscles on the first day after birth, even though the belly will probably feel quite flabby.

1. Lie flat on back (on bed or floor), with knees bent.

2. Place fingertips of one hand in the center of belly just below the navel and gently press in.

3. Raise head, bringing chin to chest as far toward the breasts as possible. With your fingertips you will feel the abdominal muscles tightening and approaching the middle of the belly from either side.

   If your muscles are in extremely good tone, they will come together at the midline. But more likely, you will feel a soft spot in between the right and left abdominal muscles.

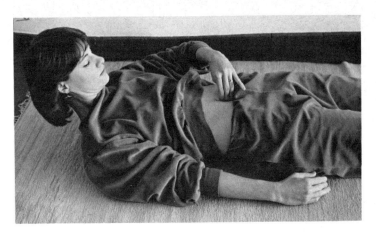

Checking for separation of the abdominal muscles

Notice how wide this spot is. If wide, you will be able to put several fingers in between the two tight bands of muscle.

Work on decreasing the degree of separation with the following "Chin-to-Chest" exercise. Meanwhile, avoid alternate knee curl-ups, or exercises requiring twisting the hips and rotating the trunk, until the separation is corrected.

CHIN-TO-CHEST

In her classic text, *Nurse-Midwifery,* Helen Varney recommends this exercise for bringing separated abdominal muscles together. It is actually the same movement used to check for separation of the abdominal muscles.

1. Lie flat on back, with knees bent so feet are flat on the bed or floor and arms to the side.

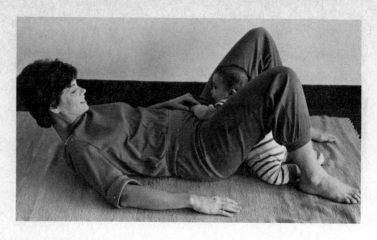

Chin-to-chest

2. Slowly bring chin to chest as far forward toward the breasts as possible (as if you were trying to put your chin between your breasts).

3. Hold for a few seconds.

4. Slowly lower head to starting position.

5. Repeat 5–10 times, once or twice daily.

The number of times and the degree the head is raised can be increased a little each day.

LEG SLIDING
This exercise is good for toning the abdominal region.

1. Lie flat on back with knees bent and feet flat on the floor or bed.

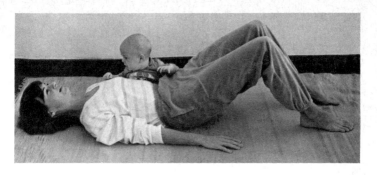

Leg sliding

2. As you breathe out, tighten the abdominal and buttock muscles, pressing back firmly against the floor or bed.

3. Slide both feet forward as far as you are able without allowing back to arch.

4. Repeat 5–10 times.

Don't be concerned if at first you are only able to slide a few inches before your back begins to arch. Keep at it. You will gradually be able to increase the distance.

HEAD AND NECK ROLLING

This exercise relaxes the head and neck muscles, which tend to become tense in nursing mothers.

1. Sitting cross-legged on the floor, drop head forward, chin toward chest, letting all the muscles of the neck go limp.

2. Roll head in a gentle circle to the left all the way around to the starting position.

3. Repeat 2–3 times.

4. Reverse direction.

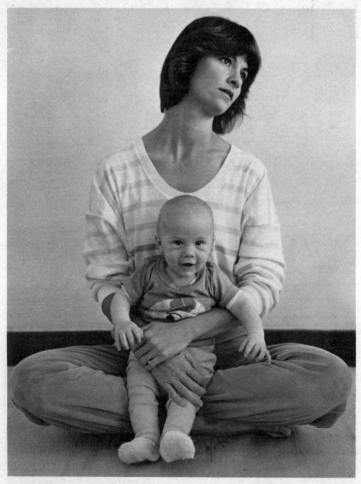

Head and neck rolling

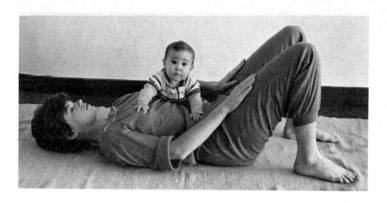

Pelvic rocking

PELVIC ROCKING

Pelvic rocking promotes greater flexibility of the back, eases backache, and improves the posture—compromised as a result of a changing center of gravity and the effect of hormones during pregnancy.

If you combine this exercise with abdominal tightening, pelvic rocking can be a back strengthener as well as an abdominal exercise. You can also add pelvic-floor contractions and work on three areas at the same time.

PELVIC ROCKING IN THE BACK-LYING POSITION

1. Lie flat on back, with feet slightly apart and knees bent. Allow entire body to relax completely.

2. Squeeze buttocks together, lifting them slightly. At the same time breathe out, tightening abdominal muscles and pushing the back flat on the floor or bed.

3. Return to starting position, relaxing abdominal muscles and buttocks.

4. Continue rocking pelvis in a gentle rocking motion for a minute or so.

When you are familiar with the motion, you can coordinate this exercise with pelvic-floor contractions, drawing up the pelvic floor as you tighten the abdominals.

Variation
This variation is a gentle abdominal and pelvic-floor exercise.

1. Hold the buttocks, abdominals, and pelvic-floor muscles with back pressed firmly to the bed or floor for a count of five.

2. Return to starting position.

3. Repeat 10–20 times.

PELVIC ROCKING ON ALL FOURS
In this position the postpartum abdomen will probably sag. More effort is required to tighten the abdominal muscles and keep the back straight.

1. Rest on all fours, palms under shoulders and back parallel to the floor. (Do not allow back to curve.)

2. Exhale and lower chin to chest, tightening buttocks and abdominal muscles as you raise lower

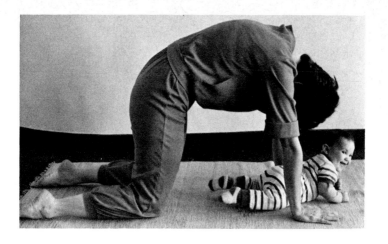

Pelvic rocking on all fours

back like an angry cat. (You can tighten the pelvic floor at the same time.)

3. Inhale, lift head, roll pelvis back, and return the back to a straightened position without letting it sag. Relax belly and pelvic floor.

4. Repeat, rocking pelvis slowly and rhythmically for a minute or so.

CURL-UPS

Do curl-ups slowly and smoothly rather than with the sudden jerky movements that result from spurts of effort. If you find this abdominal exercise difficult, do abdominal tightening or chin-to-chest until you are able to do curl-ups smoothly.

1. Lie flat on back, with knees bent and hands resting on thighs.

2. Inhale and press lower back to the floor.

3. Exhale and raise head, chin to chest and shoulders 6–8 inches off the floor, as you slide hands toward knees.

4. Hold for a count of five.

5. Lower to starting position as you inhale.

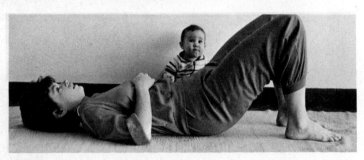

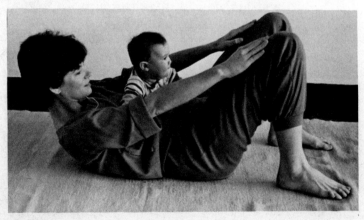

Curl-ups

6. Repeat 5–20 times. Increase the number of times as you gain strength.

Once the baby has head control, you can put him on your abdomen while doing curl-ups.

ALTERNATE KNEE CURL-UPS
Wait until you have decreased the degree of abdominal muscle separation before doing this exercise.

1. Exhale and raise head, chin to chest and shoulders off the floor, turning slightly to the left as you cross right hand over to outside of left knee.

2. Hold for a few seconds, breathing gently.

3. Lower back as you inhale.

4. Alternate sides and repeat 5–10 times on each side.

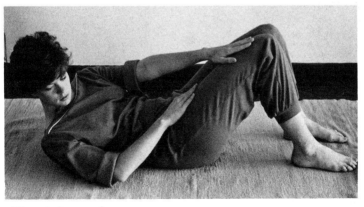

Alternate knee curl-ups

ANKLE REACHING

This exercise strengthens the abdominal muscles, slims the waist, and contributes to spinal flexibility.

1. Lie on back, with knees bent and feet flat on the floor.

2. Pull in your abdominal muscles, lifting head and shoulders slightly off the floor.

3. Bend to the left side at the waist, reaching toward left ankle as if you were going to grasp the ankle in your hand.

   Don't stretch to the point of discomfort. You probably will not be able to touch your ankle.

4. Return to starting position.

5. Do the same on the right side.

6. Repeat 5–20 times.

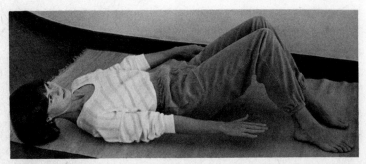

Ankle reaching

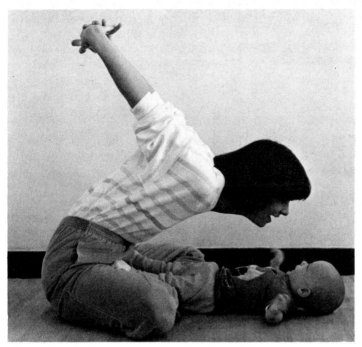

Chest expansion

CHEST EXPANSION

Especially relaxing for nursing mothers who often sit hunched over with their babies for several hours a day, this simple exercise stretches the pectoral muscles and loosens the muscles of the neck, shoulders, and upper back.

1. Sit cross-legged on the floor.

2. Clasp hands behind back.

3. Bend forward slowly and gently, raising arms as high as you can without straining. (With prac-

tice you will probably be able to touch your head to the floor. But don't try it if uncomfortable.)

4. Hold for 5–10 seconds.

5. Slowly lower arms, returning to starting position.

6. Repeat 2–3 times.

You can also do this exercise in a standing position:

1. With hands clasped behind back, gently bend forward, lowering head toward thighs and raising arms, only as far as you can without straining.

2. Hold for 5–10 seconds.

3. Slowly return to starting position, lowering arms.

THE WINDMILL

This body stretch exercises the abdominals and upper thighs.

1. Stand with feet shoulder-width apart, knees slightly flexed, and arms outstretched on either side.

2. Bend at waist and touch left hand to right foot.

3. Return to starting position.

4. Bend again, touching right hand to left foot.

5. Repeat 5–10 times, alternating sides.

Increase number of times as comfortable.

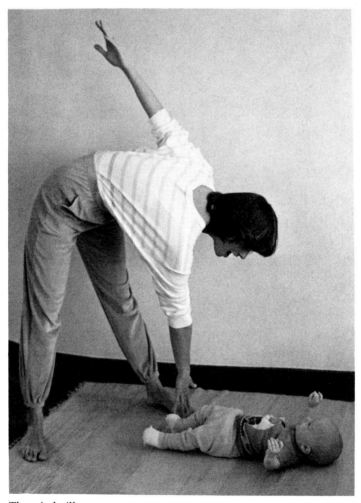

The windmill

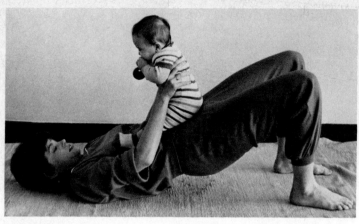

The bridge

THE BRIDGE

"The Bridge" strengthens the lower back and the abdominal and buttock muscles and contributes to spinal flexibility.

1. Lie flat on back, with feet slightly apart and knees bent.

2. Slowly raise buttocks and lower back off the floor, vertebra by vertebra. Don't lunge. (You can also contract pelvic-floor muscles as you raise back off the floor.) The shoulders, neck, and arms should be relaxed and remain on the floor, and there should be a straight line from shoulders to knees. Don't exaggerate the spine's natural curvature.

3. Hold for a few seconds.

4. Exhale and slowly lower the back, one vertebra at a time.

5. Gently press the lower back to the floor and draw belly in.

6. Repeat 2–3 times.

You can do this with your baby on your abdomen once he has head control.

ROWING

Rowing exercises the abdominal muscles and back.

1. Sit up with knees bent in front of you.

2. Stretch arms straight out as if you were rowing a boat.

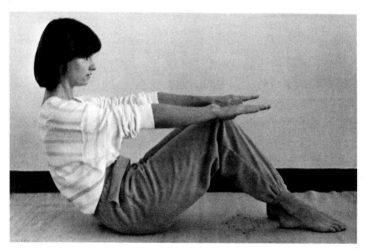

Rowing

3. Slowly curl back until your back is about half-way to the floor.

4. Stop. Hold for a count of five.

5. Slowly return to starting position.

6. Repeat 5–10 times.

WALKING ON THE BUTTOCKS

This rather odd-looking exercise helps slim the waist as it strengthens the back, abdominal region, and thighs.

Your baby can sit on your thighs as you do buttocks-walking.

1. Sit on the floor with back erect and legs straight in front of you.

2. Tighten abdominal muscles and take six sliding steps forward on your buttocks.

3. Return to starting position, "walking" backward on your buttocks.

4. Repeat 5–10 times.

BACK-LYING WAIST TWIST

This exercise trims the waist as it stretches and relaxes the back.

1. Lie flat on back, with knees bent and arms outstretched on either side, palms facing downward.

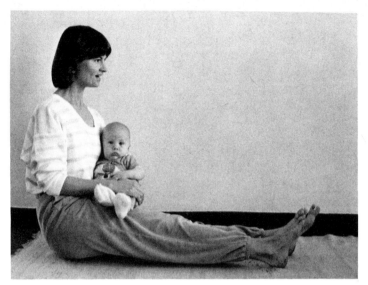

Walking on the buttocks

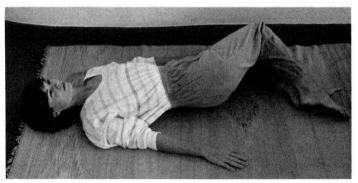

Back-lying waist twist

2. Keeping knees together and shoulders on the floor, twist from waist, swinging both knees to the left until they touch or nearly touch the floor.

3. Return to starting position. Swing knees to the right.

4. Repeat 5–20 times.

RELAXATION

The need for relaxation is especially great during the postpartum period. Tension-causing events—the baby's constant demands and crying, your own concerns—are at an all-time high. Excessive tension, however, can contribute to fatigue, irritability, depression, and possibly nursing problems.

End each exercise session with physical and mental relaxation.

The following "progressive relaxation" exercise is most effective for teaching your body the difference between tense and relaxed muscles and for bringing about a state of complete physical relaxation.

Remove shoes. If you wear glasses, remove them also. Wear comfortable, loose clothing and do the exercise in a warm, dimly lit room.

Your partner or friend can read the instructions to you in a soft voice as you do the exercise. He should pause between each step, giving you time to complete the step before going on.

Or, you can read through the instructions, then do the exercise. You'll find that it gets a little easier each time you try it.

Take your time. Once you feel you are aware of the difference between tension and relaxation, you will no longer have to tense and release each muscle group individually. You can simply let your awareness travel through your body, telling yourself to relax.

1. Lie in any comfortable position on the bed or floor, using pillows wherever you wish. Many find this exercise easier in the back-lying position.

2. Take a deep breath so that the abdomen *rises on the in breath* and *falls on the out breath.*

   As you begin to relax, let your breathing become just a little deeper and a little slower than usual without straining.

3. Now tighten the muscles of left arm and hand, clenching your fist. Hold for a few seconds.

   Release, letting arm and hand go limp.

   Feel the relaxation in your arm and hand.

4. Tighten the muscles of right arm and hand, clenching your fist. Hold for a few seconds.

   Release, letting arm and hand go limp.

   Feel the relaxation in your arm and hand.

   For the next few minutes, each time you release a muscle group take a few seconds to feel the relaxation.

5. Tighten the muscles of left leg and foot, curling the toes.

Release, letting leg and foot go limp.

6. Tighten the muscles of right leg and foot, curl ing the toes.

   Release, letting leg and foot go limp.

7. Squeeze buttocks together tightly.

   Release.

8. Draw up the muscles of pelvic floor.

   Release.

9. Arch the back slightly.

   Release, letting the muscles of your back become completely relaxed.

10. Tighten shoulders by pushing them back as if you were trying to make the shoulder blades touch one another.

    Release, letting shoulders fall limp.

11. Tighten the muscles of neck by arching neck slightly as if you were trying to look up.

    Release, letting neck fall limp.

12. Clench teeth together, tightening the muscles of jaw.

    Release.

13. Squint your eyes.

    Release, letting eyelids fall heavy.

14. Furrow the brow.

   Release, letting the space between the eyes feel as if it is getting wider.

15. Now take a few deep breaths.

   Allow your breathing to become a little slower, a little deeper than usual without straining in any way.

   Feel the breath filling the abdominal region, the middle chest, and finally the upper chest.

   Feel any additional tension melting away as you exhale.

16. Let your awareness travel through your body.

   If you find any areas that could be more re-laxed, feel the tension melt away as you breathe out.

17. When you are ready, open your eyes and gen-tly stretch.

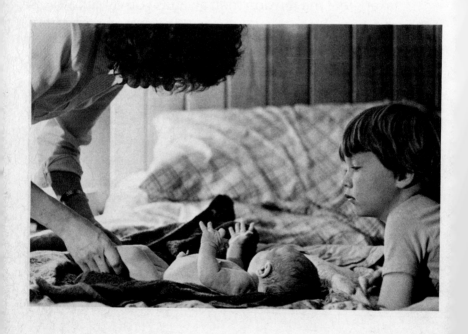

chapter six
· · · · · · · ·

After a cesarean birth

The majority of cesarean deliveries are unplanned. For most cesarean mothers, the decision to have surgery comes as a surprise. Many have never even considered the possibility of having surgery.

Of course, if you do know in advance that you are going to have a cesarean birth, you can prepare yourself by taking special cesarean classes and gathering as much information as possible. Taking these preliminary steps will reduce anxiety considerably and pave the way for a smoother postpartum recovery.

Once the decision to do a cesarean is made, the mother may react in various ways. Many are disappointed. Some mothers are too stunned or exhausted to react until after birth. Some women are relieved that labor will finally be over and they will soon see their babies—particularly if it has been a long labor. After Jane had spent nearly two days in labor and several hours in fruitless pushing, her sympathetic obstetrician reluctantly suggested a cesarean. Though tears of frustration welled in Jane's eyes, she consented willingly. "At that point I just wanted to get the whole thing over with quickly."

Paula and her husband, John, had not been in the hospital for more than twelve hours when their physician suggested a cesarean. The mother's labor had failed to progress. Though there was no emergency and Paula could have simply waited for her labor to pick up again, the idea of surgery didn't seem to bother her. John was equally matter-of-fact. "Oh well, I'm sure the doctor knows his business. We'll just flow along with the tide."

However, for those who have hoped, planned, and prepared for a natural birth, the decision to do a cesarean can be devastating. As one mother said about her surgical birth, "It was emotionally difficult to accept the reality of it after all those months of planning." One mother who opted for a cesarean after trying unsuccessfully to turn her breech baby said, "It was an incredible disappointment—a change in all the plans we had made up to that point."

Many fathers are intensely sad and perhaps outraged when the decision to do surgery is made. David, one expectant father, was asked to remain in the waiting room until after his partner was prepped for the operation. There he collapsed in a chair, his elbows on his knees, holding his head in his hands, looking like a man who had just lost his only child. "I can hardly believe this is happening," he said with tears in his eyes.

Fear is an almost inevitable accompaniment to cesarean birth, even if the parents are well prepared. Most mothers are frightened about the surgery, most fathers worried about their partner. Among the biggest fears are of the unknown and of being out of control. During a natural birth, the mother actively participates. She is involved in a normal life process. Ideally, her caregiver is present only to assist her. During a cesarean, on the other hand, everything is different. The mother does not give birth actively. She is operated on. Though she may participate in certain decisions—about what medication to take, the type of anesthesia she will have, and so forth—her sense of control is gone. She is entirely in the hands of her physician.

Though cesarean surgery should certainly be avoided when possible, an unavoidable cesarean need not be a negative experience.

Cynthia and Dan, for example, made their cesarean birth as positive as possible. They had prepared for a natural birth, but on the day labor began discovered that the baby was breech. Their obstetrician planned to deliver the baby vaginally, but Cynthia's cervix did not fully dilate after many long hours of labor.

Making the decision jointly with the physician, the parents opted for a cesarean birth. "I felt relieved," Cynthia recalls, "just knowing the baby would be healthy.

"Dan helped me immensely," she continued. "He watched the delivery and held my hand, telling me what was going on so I could relax."

After the birth, Cynthia fell into a deep sleep as a result of morphine and the exhaustion from a long labor. "I woke to find the baby nursing at my breast, Dan standing nearby, supporting him."

The mother remained in the hospital only three days. During that time Dan slept in the same room with her and the baby. "The baby never went to the nursery. One of us was with him every minute."

Afterward, Cynthia was sad that she had needed surgery. "I had wanted to deliver normally and felt somewhat robbed. For a while I was worried that if I got pregnant again I might have to have another C-section. Now I no longer have that fear, since I've talked to so many women who have had vaginal births after cesareans."

A world of difference separates cesarean from normal, natural birth. Yet fortunately, there is also a world of difference between cesarean surgery and any other operation.

A child is born.

THE RISING CESAREAN RATE
Cesarean surgery has saved the lives of many mothers and babies. In rare cases, a cesarean birth can be a welcome intervention. However, in the United States the cesarean rate has reached outrageous proportions. The percentage of surgical deliveries has quadrupled since 1969. In 1985, it was an appalling 20 percent! This means that one in every five mothers gives birth via major abdominal surgery. In some hospitals the cesarean rate is even higher—30 percent, even 40 percent!

The mother's body was aptly designed to give birth naturally and normally. Few but the most fanatic would deny that. Why, then, is our cesarean rate so high?

A number of reasons can be cited, reflecting both genuine complications and a changing American attitude toward birth. It is important for the mother to be aware of these reasons before birth, so that she can take steps to avoid unnecessary surgery.

INDICATIONS FOR A CESAREAN BIRTH

The decision to do nearly 80 percent of all cesarean births is made as a result of one or more of the following: prolonged labor, CPD (cephalopelvic disproportion, a condition in which the baby's head is supposedly too large for the mother's pelvis); breech birth; fetal distress; and previous cesarean section. However, as many childbirth professionals have pointed out, these are not always unavoidable reasons for cesarean surgery.

CPD is perhaps the most often-cited reason for doing a cesarean. Genuine CPD is an extremely rare condition. Even when the suspicion that the mother's pelvis is too small is confirmed by X-ray, CPD is not necessarily an indication for surgery. The bones in the baby's head mold to the shape of the pelvis during labor. In addition, the pelvic bone's structure allows some "play" as a result of hormones that relax the ligaments (tough connective tissue that holds the bones together) in preparation for childbearing.

In their hard-hitting book, *Silent Knife*, Nancy Wainer Cohen and Lois J. Estner tell the stories of several mothers who had cesarean sections because of CPD, yet later gave birth to *larger* babies vaginally. One mother birthed a "10 pound 6 ounce baby two years after being sectioned for her 7 pound baby."[1] Several other mothers who'd had cesareans for CPD in hospitals later gave birth to larger babies at home.

Fetal distress is the cause of most cesareans labeled "emergency." Yet this is often an avoidable condition.

Fetal distress can be precipitated by injudicious use of medication and unnecessary medical intervention, as well as prolonged maternal anxiety. For example, studies have linked the use of electronic fetal monitoring with a rise as high as three times in the cesarean rate, with no improvement in fetal outcome.[2, 3] (The electronic fetal monitor was originally devised for use with high-risk labors. However, electronic monitoring has since become routine procedure in many hospitals.) Some believe that the monitor creates the very problems—fetal distress and complications of labor—that it was designed to detect!

Actually, this is not so surprising as it seems. If the mother is continuously monitored, she is relatively immobile. This is all the more true if she has internal monitoring, in which case a wire passes up the vagina, through the cervix, and is attached to the fetus's scalp. Freedom to move around, walk around the corridors, walk outside if she wishes, and to enjoy whatever activity feels normal for her is one of the best ways to assist labor in progressing naturally. The monitored woman is prohibited this freedom.

More importantly, electronic monitoring—and, for that matter, all avoidable medical intervention including intravenous feeding—may precipitate psychological distress at a time when the mother is particularly vulnerable. This in turn may affect the mother's labor and contribute to fetal distress.

Previous surgical delivery is another common indication for cesarean surgery. Many obstetricians elect to do repeat cesareans. This practice, however, is fortunately changing, and more and more physicians are realizing that a large percentage of women who have given birth surgically in the past are as likely to have normal vaginal births as other mothers.

Other indications for cesarean surgery include: prolonged labor or failure to progress in labor; unfavorable fetal position in the uterus; prolapsed cord (a rare condition in which the umbilical cord slips down into the birth canal before the baby); *placenta previa* (the placenta lying over the cervix); *abruptio placenta* (placental detachment from the uterine wall); and maternal disease such as herpes, diabetes, or eclampsia.

The major underlying reason the American cesarean rate is so high, I believe, is that many American health professionals and parents alike tend to view birth as a medical event rather than a natural, normal part of life. Mothers are often separated from their families, isolated in hospitals, and treated like invalids. This cannot fail to interrupt what would otherwise be a perfectly natural event.

Though there is a widespread movement toward natural birth, birth at home and in childbearing centers, an opposite pull is felt in the direction of increased technological intervention. Hospitals, for the most part, are becoming better places to give birth—not only safer but more comfortable. Humanistic maternity care is increasingly available. Yet in some hospitals, birth is still viewed almost as if it were a pathological process. Healthy laboring women are still being hooked up to routine intravenous feeding and are being treated as though they were ill.

This by no means implies that all cesareans are avoidable. But a large percentage—perhaps the overwhelming majority—can be avoided.

PREVENTING AN UNNECESSARY CESAREAN

No couple living in a country with the phenomenally high surgical birth rate of the United States can afford to overlook preventive measures. Every couple—whether planning to birth at home, in a childbearing center, or in a hospital—should take steps to minimize the chance of surgery.

If you observe preventive measures and nevertheless do have a cesarean, at least you know that you have done all you could to avoid *unnecessary* surgery. This is a long step in lessening the negative emotions that so often follow cesarean delivery.

The following steps will increase your chance of birthing normally:

BEFORE BIRTH

• Eat a nutritious, well-balanced diet throughout pregnancy. Studies have shown that a mother's prenatal diet has much to do with whether or not her birth is normal.

• Exercise regularly.

• Choose a caregiver with a low cesarean rate.

• Choose a comfortable birthing environment.

• Seek another opinion if you are told in advance that you *must* give birth by cesarean section.

IN LABOR

• Drink fluids and eat lightly as you feel the need.

• Avoid the flat-on-the-back position, which can lead to fetal distress.

• Avoid routine medical intervention—artificial rupture of the membranes, intravenous feeding, and continuous electronic fetal monitoring, all of which can impair labor.

• Avoid pain medication if possible. Try nonpharmacological means of pain relief first. (See *Sharing Birth: A Father's Guide to Giving Support During Labor* for suggestions the father can use to reduce the pain and in some cases the length of labor.)

VAGINAL BIRTH AFTER CESAREAN

The old dictum "Once a cesarean, always a cesarean" is no longer recognized as valid. In fact, vaginal birth after a cesarean is in most cases safer than repeat surgery.

If you plan a vaginal birth after a previous cesarean, find a caregiver wholly supportive of your plans. Be sure to choose a caregiver who will treat you like a normal, healthy woman, not as if you were doing something dangerous. Being treated like an invalid through labor will decrease your chances of birthing naturally. Though careful observation is wise, you should not be prevented from using a birthing room or be required to have continuous electronic fetal monitoring.

For further information on preventing unnecessary cesareans, see the list of resources at the end of this book.

THE FIRST FEW HOURS

Cesarean surgery takes about an hour. But birth will probably occur during the first fifteen minutes. The remaining time is spent stitching the incision.

Though cesarean delivery has definite drawbacks, it is still birth. A baby is born and a woman and man have become mother and father. The joy and awe that usually accompany the childbearing miracle may flood over you both when you first greet the child—regardless of the fact that you are in an operating room being stitched. Assuming the baby is healthy, the matchless emotion that crowns human birth is as real for cesarean parents as for those who have birthed vaginally.

Two basic types of anesthesia are used for cesarean surgery: *general anesthesia*, in which case the mother is unconscious; and *regional anesthesia*, in which she is anesthetized but awake. Most mothers prefer the latter so they are able to experience the birth and greet the baby as soon as it is born.

Regional anesthesia may be either a *spinal* or *epidural*. Both are administered by means of a needle in the back. In the epidural, a hollow tube is left in the back for the duration of surgery so that more anesthesia can be injected as needed. Epidural anesthesia does not penetrate the *dura*, the thick outer covering of the spinal cord. Spinal anesthesia does. Sometimes, with a spinal, a small amount of cerebrospinal fluid is lost, resulting later in a *spinal headache*.

Both types of regional anesthesia numb the body from chest to toes and render that area temporarily immobile. Though you may feel pressure, tugging, and pulling during surgery, there should be no pain. If there is, simply tell the physician so the anesthesia can be adjusted.

It is best for you, your partner, and your child to remain together in the operating room as long as the baby is healthy. If born prematurely or with other complications requiring immediate medical care, the baby may be taken to an intensive care unit for special attention. Your partner can either remain with you for the duration of the surgery or go to the nursery with the newborn. You can request to be wheeled to the nursery after the operation is complete. But under most circumstances there is no reason you and your child should have to be separated.

The father has an especially important role during and immediately after surgical delivery. Ideally, he should remain at his partner's side throughout the birth. As I point out in my previous book, *Sharing Birth: A Father's Guide to Giving Support During Labor*, the father's invaluable presence during surgery will make the mother feel more secure and more as if she is participating in a birth rather than merely being operated on.

The father does not have to witness the surgery. A screen placed between the mother's head and abdomen blocks both parents' views. Of course, if he wants to witness the actual birth, he can simply stand up.

The father of triplets delivered via cesarean section enthusiastically recalls: "I witnessed the entire thing. It was fantastic watching the delivery of three babies!"

Another father said, "I didn't want to stay seated behind the screen. So I stood and observed. For a moment I didn't think I was going to make it through watching the operation. But when the obstetrician pulled the baby out, it was wonderful!"

Today, most hospitals recognize a father's right to attend the birth of his child, whether that birth takes place vaginally or surgically. Since the decision to do cesarean surgery most often comes unexpectedly during labor, choosing a hospital that encourages the father's presence in the delivery room is vitally important. This decision should be made during pregnancy even if you plan to give birth at home—just in case of a last-minute transfer. Couples are strongly urged to avoid any hospital that does not endorse the father's presence at cesarean birth.

For the hospital staff and obstetrician, cesarean surgery is a common procedure. For the mother, however, though the surgery is safe, it is anything but routine.

If you are like most women, you will probably be frightened. The father's presence and emotional support can ease anxiety tremendously. Just holding his partner's hand and sharing the tense moments before the child is born can make all the difference in the world.

Immediately after birth, while the physician stitches the incision, the father's most important task (provided that there are no complications) is to hold the baby. He should hold it close to the mother so they both can see the newborn. The mother's hands may not be free, but the father can hold the baby close enough for her to caress the baby with her face. Kissing her child, making eye contact, and smelling the fresh odor of her newborn will be a wonderful beginning to motherhood.

With his hand cupped over the baby's eyes, the father can shield the newborn from bright light. This way both parents can enjoy eye contact with the child even though the room will not be dimly lit. (No physician, however progressive, will do surgery in the dark!)

If you and your baby are separated immediately after birth, you can make up for this time either in the recovery room or later in the postpartum room. Initiating breastfeeding as soon as you are able and spending as much time as possible with your baby will smooth out this rocky beginning. If the separation is prolonged as a result of prematurity or other complications, you can make up for this at home.

In The Recovery Room

Shortly after surgery, you will be taken to a recovery room for two or three hours, or until the anesthesia has worn off and your condition stabilized. The recovery room stay may be somewhat longer in some hospitals, depending on your condition and available nursing staff. In other hospitals, mothers are taken right from surgery to the postpartum floor. In some hospitals, cesarean mothers recover along with other surgical patients. The latter situation is to be avoided if possible, as the father will not be permitted to remain with you should there be several patients in one room.

Wherever you recover, during your first few hours after surgery a nurse will check your temperature, pulse, blood pressure, respiration, vaginal discharge, and the incision site. You may also be given a bed bath, toothbrush, and mouthwash to freshen up.

During this initial recovery period and later in the postpartum room, a nurse will periodically check your uterus with a hand on your abdomen to make sure it remains contracted. The uterus should remain well contracted to prevent hemorrhage at the placental site (see pages 23–28). The pressure of her manual exam may be painful. If so, don't be afraid to ask her to be more gentle.

Pitocin may be added to the IV bottle. This hormonal preparation stimulates uterine contractions. If after-birth contractions are painful, ask for medication.

What happens in the recovery room depends on the type of anesthesia used. If you have had general anesthesia, you may feel quite groggy at first. In the case of regional, a nurse will probably ask you to wiggle your toes, move your feet, and bend your knees as soon as possible. After a spinal, you may have to remain flat on your back for eight to twelve hours to prevent head-ache.

As the anesthesia wears off, your legs may begin to tingle for a while. This may feel odd, but will not be painful. You also may feel discomfort (ranging from mild to painful) and/or a burning sensation at the incision site. Pain medication will mitigate discomfort.

Concerning her recovery room experience, Renee re-calls: "I was very excited, but the medication caused me to have trouble thinking clearly. It required enormous effort to put my thoughts together and express them. I didn't feel myself for about ten hours, and consequently didn't feel much involved with the baby."

Pain-relief medication may make you feel drowsy. You may just want to go to sleep. One new mother, Janet, can barely recall the time she spent in the recovery room. "I don't remember anything. I was too drowsy and spaced out. All I wanted to do was to go to sleep, even though I knew it would be a drag for my husband Bill to sit there and watch me snore."

Another mother, whose second child was born via cesarean section due to a condition of active herpes, said, "I felt gypped. As it turned out, I had general anesthesia. My first memory when I woke was of my husband standing nearby, pointing to the baby in the incubator. I remember thinking 'I do love her.' But I couldn't take her right then. I just wanted to go back to sleep."

On the other hand, like some mothers you may be so relieved that labor is over and so elated with the baby that sleep is the farthest thing from your mind. As Carolyn said after the cesarean birth of her first child, a

7 ½ lb. girl, "I was so excited! I talked constantly to my husband. When he went out of the room for a few minutes to announce the news to the grandparents, I kept up a steady stream of conversation with the nurses."

If you and your partner are like most parents, and if you're not too tired, you'll probably want to share the news with relatives and friends minutes after birth. This is a good time to make phone calls should there be a phone in the recovery room. If not, you may have to wait until you get to the postpartum unit.

Provided the baby is healthy and you are awake and aware, this is a good time to be with the baby and enjoy the ongoing process of parent-infant attachment. The normal course of the maternal-infant relationship has received a traumatic shock thanks to surgery. If mother and baby have been separated—often the case after cesarean birth—they should be reunited as soon as possible. Being together in the recovery room—you, your partner, and baby—will give your new family the best possible start.

Initiate breastfeeding. The nurse or father can help tremendously. Don't worry about medication getting to the baby. The amount secreted through the mother's milk is minimal. But it is important for the baby to get the benefits of colostrum (see pages 11–12) and be snuggled at the breast.

Most cesarean mothers experience a mixture of feelings in the recovery room: relief that the surgery is over, discomfort, and joy about the birth. Regardless of how you have delivered, you and your baby are together. For now, that is the really important thing.

THE FIRST FEW DAYS:
IN THE POSTPARTUM ROOM

The average hospital stay after cesarean birth is three to seven days. If you wish an early discharge, discuss it with your physician. You may be able to arrange to leave within two or three days after surgery. If so, you might consider hiring a postpartum helper to assist at home, unless your partner is able to be with you throughout the day.

After surgery, the IV and catheter will remain in for twenty-four to forty-eight hours. The IV provides nourishment and fluid until the intestines begin to function. The catheter keeps the bladder empty until you are able to get up and urinate.

At first your diet will probably consist of liquids. You will gradually move toward a regular diet.

While you remain in the hospital, a nurse will continue to check your vital signs (temperature, pulse, blood pressure, and respiration), the dressing, and your uterus to make sure it remains contracted. A discharge of lochia will follow cesarean birth, just as it does vaginal birth. You may wish to wear beltless pads. (Lochia is discussed on pages 26–28.)

Ordinary activities—walking, coughing, sneezing, laughing—will be uncomfortable for a while. Don't hesitate to ask for medication if you feel the need.

While still in bed, wiggle your toes to stimulate circulation.

A nurse will probably ask you to do deep breathing, coughing, or huffing to clear the lungs of the excess mucus that tends to accumulate after surgery. Coughing or huffing helps prevent pneumonia. Simply take a deep breath and exhale with an audible "huff." A towel or pillow pressed firmly against the incision will ease discomfort.

No doubt after surgery the last thing you'll want to do is exercise! Yet the cesarean mother's first exercises—besides wiggling the toes and coughing or huffing—should begin on the very first postpartum day.

Shift your position in bed often. This will become less uncomfortable with practice. Moving about facilitates blood circulation, promotes healing, helps prevent postsurgical complications such as phlebitis (inflammation of a vein), and decreases the likelihood of gas pains.

Begin abdominal-tightening exercise the first postoperative day. This very simple exercise will both strengthen the muscles and help prevent gas pains.

1. Take a deep breath so that the belly rises on the in breath. Breathe out evenly and steadily, tightening the abdominal muscles as much as possible on the out breath (as if you were trying to make your abdominal wall touch your spine).

2. Repeat 4–5 times every hour. Don't worry about the incision. It will not come apart.

Following are some additional exercises that you can do while still in bed:

Foot bending and circling. (See pages 97–98.) These will stimulate circulation in the lower extremities and help prevent *thrombosis* (the formation of a blood clot). You needn't continue this exercise once you are out of bed.

Pelvic rocking in the back-lying position. (See pages 107–8.) Accompany this exercise with gentle tightening

141 · *After a cesarean birth*

of the abdominal muscles to promote healing of the incision and encourage intestinal activity.

Once you are at home and feeling stronger, you can do the same postpartum exercises as the woman who has delivered vaginally. It will, however, take more time for you to strengthen and firm up the belly, since the abdominal muscles have been severed. You will, of course, also require more rest at first.

Consult your caregiver before beginning an exercise program. Many caregivers prefer that new mothers wait until after their six-week checkup to begin strenuous exercises. Meanwhile, deep breathing, abdominal tightening, Kegel exercises, and gentle arm and leg exercises can be done anytime, even in bed.

Getting Out of Bed

You should get up shortly after cesarean birth—ideally within the first twelve hours. Getting up early and walking around minimizes the chance of developing a blood clot and reduces postoperative gas pains.

The first day or two, the IV and catheter may remain in place, but this will not prevent you from walking very short distances.

A nurse will help you the first time you rise from bed. Don't attempt to do it yourself!

The first time out of bed, take it little by little. First, sit at the edge of the bed for a moment. Place your hands over the incision, pressing firmly to support it. When you get up, you may feel pulling and tugging sensations at the area around the incision. Some women imagine that the incision will pop open—a common but rather frightening thought! But this will not happen. Also, when you first stand up, you may have a sudden gush of vaginal discharge.

Many cesarean mothers automatically adopt what has been referred to as the "cesarean shuffle"—a stooping position while walking—to protect the incision and minimize discomfort. Avoid this. Try to stand tall, rather than slouched over. This will help the incision heal better. You can always lean on your partner or a nurse for support.

The first time out of bed may be very difficult and require a tremendous amount of effort. As one new cesarean mother said, "The hardest part was getting out of bed and taking the first step!" But the more you move and walk around, the easier it will become.

Rooming-In

Remaining together with your child as much as possible after birth is particularly important for the cesarean mother. Rooming-in will facilitate breastfeeding, aid in the development of the maternal-infant attachment process, and reduce postpartum depression and trauma. Though it may be uncomfortable and difficult at times, being together enables you to focus on the birth, the fact that you are beginning a family, rather than on the operation. As one new cesarean mother said, "I felt as if I were robbed out of a vaginal birth. I wasn't going to be robbed out of those early hours with my baby."

You don't have to remain together with your baby every minute if you don't want to. You may prefer partial rooming-in. If you feel you need time for yourself, tell the nurse that you would like to put the baby in the nursery for a while. As Bonnie Donovan writes in her book, *The Cesarean Birth Experience*, "The quality of the time spent with the baby is far superior to the quantity."[4]

You may find rooming-in somewhat trying at times. You will be uncomfortable from the stitches and far less mobile than the mother who has given birth vaginally. If you are like most cesarean mothers, you will probably feel especially awkward taking care of your baby. Beginning the caretaking responsibilities while recovering from major surgery puts the cesarean mother at a considerable disadvantage.

Don't hesitate to ask the nursing staff for help. A nurse can do much to help you feel more comfortable and make you more secure in your caretaking role with the baby. Above all, the person who can help most is the father. There is no substitute for his presence and help with the baby.

Siblings should also be given the opportunity to see and hold the baby as soon as possible. It is important for other children to have the freedom to spend as much time with the mother as both the mother and the children wish. (Some hospitals place restrictions on sibling visits. Couples are urged to avoid any institution that does not welcome children to be with their mother whenever desired.)

NURSING AFTER CESAREAN BIRTH

The baby born via major surgery needs mother's milk just as much as the baby born vaginally. After surgical birth, both mother and baby will benefit from the special closeness nursing affords, although nursing will be more difficult at first.

Nurse as soon after birth as possible. The recovery

room is the best place to begin. Try not to put off breastfeeding unless absolutely necessary. Until the nursing cycle is established, the more supplemental feedings a baby receives in a nursery, the more likely minor breastfeeding problems may develop.

Obviously, if you have had general anesthesia, or if the baby needs immediate medical attention, breastfeeding will have to be postponed. In this case, begin nursing whenever you are able. It is never too late.

Once nursing is initiated, many cesarean mothers choose to supplement feedings with an occasional bottle. This provides the mother with extra time to rest and may relieve the pressure of having to assume a full-time caretaking role at a time when *she* is still in need of care. Bear in mind, however, that it is best to wait until your milk supply is well established before supplementing. Supplemental feeding, especially during the first four to six weeks, may impair milk production and make the baby less eager for the breast (getting breast milk requires more work). If you do choose to supplement nursing, try to place minimal emphasis on the bottle. Above all, don't feel guilty about supplemental nursing. Breastfeeding need not be an all-or-nothing affair. It is far better to supplement nursing than not to nurse at all.

Holding the baby directly over the incision will be painful and should be avoided. Try different positions and change position as often as you want.

Side-lying. Lie on your side with the baby cradled in your arms and facing you. Use pillows to support your back, belly, and perhaps your upper leg. After nursing, you can roll over on your back and hold the baby up to burp him.

Be sure to nurse from both breasts. When you have

finished feeding from one breast, simply roll over on your other side and nurse from the other. Your partner or a nurse can help you.

Sitting. Place a pillow over the stitches before cradling the baby in your arm and nursing. Sit with bent knees to lessen strain on the abdomen. The hospital bed can be cranked up to a comfortable position.

Football hold. While sitting up, hold your baby with your hand firmly under his head, as if you were holding a football.

If your IV interferes with breastfeeding, don't hesitate to ask to have it changed to allow maximum movement. Ask that the IV be placed in the weaker arm and in the veins of the forearm, rather than on the inner arm at the elbow. If these veins are too small, the hand is preferable to the elbow.

THE CESAREAN MOTHER'S SPECIAL NEEDS

The cesarean mother is in a unique situation. She must recover both from having given birth and from major abdominal surgery. In the hospital and later at home, she must meet the needs of her baby while developing a maternal-infant relationship. For any new mother, this is an emotionally and physically exhausting experience. For the cesarean mother, it is even more so.

Both mother and baby are compromised after surgical birth. At birth, mother and baby are dependent on each other for their physical and emotional well-being. The baby needs to be held, caressed, nursed, and loved as soon as it is born. The mother also needs the baby at this time. The baby's suckling at the breast, as mentioned earlier, stimulates uterine contractions, which in turn deliver the placenta and help prevent postpartum hemorrhage.

She needs the baby for her emotional well-being as well. She has carried her child as an inner presence, a real and living part of herself, for nine months. Throughout pregnancy, her entire body and emotions have been nurturing the baby and preparing to continue nurturing her child. Early maternal-infant separation is perhaps the major cause of postpartum depression (see pages 54–55).

After cesarean birth, however, the baby is often taken to a special-care nursery for twelve to twenty-four hours, while the mother is left to be cared for by the nursing staff. In the not-too-distant past, all were taken to a special-care nursery because of the high incidence of prematurity and respiratory distress among cesarean babies. Though this is changing, a few hospitals still may routinely remove the baby from the mother.

The cesarean mother is all but helpless. She and her partner can, of course, request that the baby remain with them unless there are serious medical complications requiring special attention. Yet she still must submit to hospital policy.

After a vaginal birth, on the other hand, if the mother doesn't like a particular policy, she can get up and go home, taking her baby with her. A nurse recently told me a story about a mother who delivered naturally in a busy hospital. Immediately after birth, the nurse left the room for a few minutes to get eye drops for the newborn. When she returned, the mother and baby had vanished! What's most remarkable is that the mother was wearing only a hospital johnnie fully open at the back! This is a somewhat extreme case, but it does indicate the great freedom of the mother who has birthed normally.

As mentioned before, most new mothers feel dependent on others, especially during the first twenty-four to forty-eight hours after birth. This phase of needing to be cared for fades as the mother recovers and establishes her own caretaking role. The cesarean mother's sense of dependence and vulnerability is magnified and prolonged. She needs special care.

Her basic needs both in the hospital and at home are, like those of all new mothers, rest, relaxation, and nurturing.

Be sure to get plenty of rest. Hospital routine—checking vital signs, bed baths, bed changes, and so forth—may make rest difficult. If you want to take a nap, tell the nurse that you don't want to be disturbed for a while. Perhaps she can hang a DO NOT DISTURB sign on your door.

Let your feelings be your guide regarding visitors. Be sure to save most of your energy and time for your baby and for getting rest. If necessary, your partner can limit the number of visitors and the length of their stay. On the other hand, you may find visitors a welcome interruption to hospital routine and perhaps boredom.

Mothering the Cesarean Mother

Taking paternity leave is vitally important after surgical birth. The father's presence is needed both in the hospital and for at least a week after discharge. The father is able to help tremendously. The simplest things will make a world of difference to the recovering mother.

He can bring the baby to the mother and help her assume a comfortable position for nursing (see pages 145–46).

Adjusting pillows and raising or lowering the bed may make the mother more comfortable. She may want him to rub her back or brush her hair.

He can remind her to do abdominal tightening and other exercises.

The father can also spend time bathing and diapering the baby, getting familiar with his own caretaking role. In addition, he can take care of the baby while the mother catches up on much-needed rest.

Above all, his presence is most important. The new parents can discuss their feelings and share their somewhat difficult beginning to parenthood.

The assistance of understanding, sensitive relatives and friends may enable the mother to feel more positive, often reducing the frustration and depression that may follow cesarean delivery.

You may also consider hiring a professional postpartum helper, especially if your partner cannot be at home with you and you have no one living nearby to help out.

COMMON DISCOMFORTS
FOLLOWING CESAREAN BIRTH

The cesarean mother is susceptible to the same discomforts as the mother who has delivered vaginally, with the exception of perineal pain. Relieving these is discussed in Chapter 4.

As a result of surgery, you may also experience additional discomfort. Don't hesitate to take pain medication if you are uncomfortable. The amount that reaches the baby via nursing is insignificant. But your comfort at this time is not. However, consult your caregiver before taking any medication, even over-the-counter preparations.

Gas Pains

Following normal birth, bowel function tends to slow down like a lazy stream after an August drought. Cesarean birth renders bowel function even slower as a result of the effects of anesthesia and the intestines having been handled during surgery and kept immobile afterward. By the second or third postpartum day, excess gas may build up, causing discomfort ranging from mild to severe.

Gail, a new cesarean mother, exclaimed: "The gas pains were the worst! But lying on my side with my knees up toward my chest helped." Pamela, another cesarean mother, was out of bed within twelve hours. She said, "Walking and drinking hot liquids helped reduce gas pains enormously."

Though uncomfortable, gas build-up is actually a positive sign, indicating that the intestines are beginning to function again.

TO RELIEVE

• Rock in a rocking chair at intervals, preferably while nursing the baby. According to a recent report in *Childbirth Educator*, post-cesarean mothers who have tried this almost never complain of gas pains.[5]
• Move around in bed. Roll from side to side.
• Walk.
• Do pelvic rocking in the back-lying position, (see pages 107–8).

- Do abdominal tightening, (see page 141).
- Lie on your left side, pull your knees up, and massage the abdomen from right to left.
- Avoid carbonated beverages, apple juice, iced drinks (though ice chips are fine), and drinking through a straw (which increases air intake). Avoid any foods that normally cause you to form gas.

If gas pains continue to bother you, your physician may prescribe an enema.

Shoulder Pain

Pain in either or both shoulders is caused by blood and air collecting under the diaphragm. The pain is referred via nerve passages to the shoulder. This will go away in two to three days as the blood and air are reabsorbed. Meanwhile, medication is the most effective relief.

AT HOME AFTER CESAREAN BIRTH

Homecoming will no doubt be a rather dramatic transition. The cesarean mother has been absent from home and perhaps from her family for a rather long time during this very sensitive period in her changing life. Actually, any time longer than twelve to twenty-four hours is a long time to be away from home when one is feeling as vulnerable and emotional as the new mother. This may contribute to baby blues and make adjusting to new parenthood more difficult for the whole family.

Going home as early as possible is the best way to make a smooth transition to new parenthood for many mothers. Some are discharged within three days and are only too glad to leave the hospital and be on familiar turf. Others, however, will benefit from a longer hospital stay.

Georgia, a physician and new cesarean mother, recalls: "I was exhausted from the surgery and the enormous number of phone calls and visitors. Because I was doing so well physically, however, my obstetrician discharged me. When I returned home I was quite upset and wished I had remained in the hospital longer. I didn't want to go back to household chores immediately. I also didn't have a support system lined up, because labor occurred three weeks early."

As mentioned earlier, once at home, the father can be a tremendous help. He should plan to take charge of household responsibilities for at least a week, preferably two.

Paulette, a new cesarean mother who was discharged on the fourth postdelivery day, said, "I needed Mark with me. Just getting around seemed impossible without him. He brought the baby when I needed to nurse, and often walked up and down the living room holding him when he was crying, while I rested."

Another cesarean mother said, "Jim helped me in the hospital and later at home. At the same time, he solidified his relationship with Zachary, learning how to handle, bathe, and dress him."

EMOTIONAL CHANGES

A wide range of normal feelings may follow a cesarean birth. Some new mothers are not particularly concerned about how they have given birth. To them the experience of birth is far less important than the fact that they have a healthy baby. A few actually welcome the idea of a planned cesarean, thereby avoiding labor.

On the other hand, many parents feel cheated during the recovery process and for days, weeks, even months afterward. Some carry the emotional scars that often accompany cesarean surgery for years. They feel disappointed that they missed the experience of normal birth. Some blame themselves, feeling guilty that they were somehow the cause of the unexpected turn of events. Mothers often feel that there is something wrong with them. "Why didn't my body work like other women's?" is a question they frequently ask themselves. Many experience anger at their physician, the hospital, or their childbirth educator, particularly if they believe the cesarean was unnecessary.

"In hindsight, I guess I should have fought," one mother, who believed her cesarean was avoidable, said. For her second birth, she hired a labor-support person to give emotional support and interface with the staff, in addition to the father. Though this labor was similar to her first, she did have a vaginal birth.

Frequently fathers also feel inadequate, that they have failed their partner, perhaps not given sufficient support.

Absurd as it may seem, friends and relatives often make thoughtless remarks to cesarean mothers, such as, "You did it the easy way!" That anyone could imagine major abdominal surgery being easier than vaginal birth seems incredible. Cesarean birth carries far greater discomfort, more emotional stress, and requires a much longer recovery period than normal birth. By no means has the cesarean mother "done it the easy way." She has it harder all around.

Many childbirth professionals are unaware of the intensity of the feelings cesarean parents often experience. Some physicians have the attitude that cesarean surgery is simply another way to have a baby. A few childbirth books support this view, leaving the cesarean mother wondering why she may be having such intensely negative feelings about her operation.

The view that all that matters is a safe birth is fading as more and more health professionals become aware of the emotional realities of birth. A healthy baby born safely and an emotionally rewarding birth experience are not mutually exclusive. In fact, for most mothers, the way they give birth matters very much. It is normal and healthy to grieve for the loss of a vaginal birth.

Discuss your feelings with your partner. Let the tears come. If you feel the need, contact a cesarean support group in your area (see the list of resources at the end of this book). Time and the fact that you do have a healthy baby will heal the wounds.

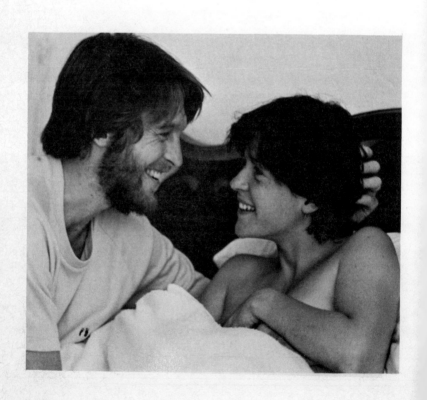

chapter seven
. . . .

Lovemaking after the baby is born

Most couples wonder when they will be able to resume lovemaking after the baby comes. There are no definite rules regarding sex that apply to all new parents. Sexual desire and comfort are individual matters.

The best thing to do is let your body be your guide about when and how to make love. How do you feel? Are you comfortable making love? Intercourse is generally safe when it is not painful. If your postpartum recovery is normal, there is no reason why you shouldn't make love whenever you want once the lochia is no longer red and the stitches from a possible tear or incision have healed.

Some physicians and midwives advise abstaining from sex until after the six-week checkup to be sure the sexual organs are healing properly and there are no complications. The six-week ban, however, is really a matter of convention and is falling by the wayside.

Four-week checkups are the rule in some practices. The French suggest waiting three weeks. Meanwhile, provided you are healthy, you can make love sooner should you desire.

Many couples have intercourse within a few days after birth. Others wait until several weeks have passed. Three weeks seems to be about average. Should you desire intercourse in less than that time, consult your caregiver for the assurance that you are healing normally.

RESUMING YOUR SEXUAL RELATIONSHIP

After the baby comes, don't expect your sexual relationship to be the same as it was before pregnancy. Though you can have sexual intercourse during the six-week postpartum recovery period, fully resuming your former relationship may take longer than six weeks. For some couples it takes several months.

Several physical and emotional factors influence the new parents' sexual relationship. The most obvious of these is the profound transformation of the mother's sexual organs during childbearing. The uterus has changed in size and shape, to say nothing of the space it occupies through pregnancy! The vagina becomes a portal wide enough for a grapefruit! One cannot expect such changes to be without effects—even if those effects are short term.

Other factors that influence lovemaking are: whether or not the mother has tears or has had an episiotomy; maternal fatigue; maternal self-image; the father's feelings; and the couple's individual needs and desires.

Normal postpartum sexual feelings vary from couple

to couple. Some find little or no change in their sex drive. They resume lovemaking very shortly after the baby comes and continue their sexual relationship without breaking stride. Others find a remarkable difference in their sexual feelings and activities. Most new mothers experience decreased sexual desire for a while.

Lela, a childbirth educator and mother of three, said, "We were making love regularly beginning three days after birth. Except for being drier for a while, I felt pretty much as I did before pregnancy." One couple said, "Lovemaking got put on hold for at least ten weeks."

After birth, especially a shared birth in which both partners actively participated, you will probably feel loving toward one another. Sharing birth can bring you closer. A new mother, Beth, recalls, "The most tender and wonderful kiss that Landon and I have ever shared was right after our daughter, Emily, was born. It felt like we had jumped into each other's skin!"

Feeling close doesn't mean you will be sexually active right away. As long as both partners' needs are met, don't be concerned. It is perfectly normal to have intercourse less often, or not at all, for several weeks. This in no way implies that your sex life is over or forever altered. It simply means that, in the words of the above-quoted couple, it is "on hold."

One or both partners may be hesitant about resuming intercourse at first. The mother may be reluctant because of discomfort, tiredness, or simply lack of desire. The father may be hesitant for fear of hurting his partner or from preoccupation with his new role. Go easily at first and tailor your lovemaking to your individual preferences.

"I was nervous about intercourse," admitted one new

mother. "I was told it was going to be very painful and that for the longest time I might not enjoy it. But it wasn't that way at all. My sexual feelings were heightened because we felt so close."

After the birth of her first child, Cheryl said: "We didn't make love for about a month. I often felt aroused when the baby was nursing, but later I didn't have a strong desire for sex. I was so sore I didn't want to be touched."

Lower maternal sexual desire is common for several weeks, and perhaps even for a few months, after the baby is born. "Of course I wouldn't deny Ted," one mother said two months after her child was born. "But I must admit my sexual desire has declined immensely." The couple should be reassured that this doesn't mean their sexual relationship is falling apart. It is simply a phase that will pass. Meanwhile, the best way to get through this period is to be open with one another, sensitive to each other's needs, and as one childbirth educator put it, "the woman generous, the man understanding."

Once resumed, the mother may respond more slowly during the first few postpartum months, without necessarily finding sexual intercourse any less satisfying. Many women want their partner to spend more time tenderly stimulating the clitoris or caressing before intercourse. Men sometimes don't realize this and have to be told. One new mother complained, "Sometimes I just got started enjoying it and it was all over."

"It may be reassuring for a woman to know that she can respond, only that it will take her longer than usual because of hormonal changes," write Elisabeth Bing and

Libby Coleman in *Making Love During Pregnancy.* "She may need extra cuddling, kissing and caressing to become aroused."[1]

Lovemaking, of course, doesn't necessarily have to include intercourse. There are other ways of showing your affection for one another and giving each other sexual fulfillment: caressing, fondling, manual stimulation of the clitoris, oral stimulation of the breasts, fellatio. Even a massage or a relaxing bath together can be quite pleasurable and a temporary substitute for making love.

Nor must you feel you have to have an orgasm every time you make love. This can lead to frustration. Not having an orgasm every time you have intercourse, especially during the first few months after birth, does not mean that something is wrong. Being less goal-oriented in your lovemaking will relieve much pressure from the need to perform. If, however, your partner feels frustrated without an orgasm, as do many men, fellatio or manual stimulation will no doubt be sexually satisfying.

If you or your partner don't feel like making love right away or if you experience minor problems at first, don't worry. Many couples think they are the only ones who experience changes in their lovemaking—and fear that these changes may be permanent. Rest assured: You are not alone. Changes in lovemaking patterns and minor problems are common after the baby is born. Most couples *do* resume their full sexual relationship in time.

Meanwhile, don't overlook aids for getting in the right mood: a glass of wine, a candlelight dinner (only after you have nursed the baby and he is off to sleep!), soft lighting, romantic music, your favorite nightgown, and so forth.

Be sure to use contraceptives if you want to prevent

another pregnancy. You may ovulate a couple of weeks before getting your first period. The hormone prolactin generally renders the ovaries inactive in a nursing mother. However, if nursing is supplemented with even an occasional bottle, the prolactin level may decrease and ovulation resume. And though unsupplemented breastfeeding makes conception unlikely until the menstrual cycle is re-established, some women nursing on demand have become pregnant. For this reason, breastfeeding cannot be trusted as a 100 percent reliable means of birth control.

Cervical caps and diaphragms are best fitted after postpartum recovery is complete. Meanwhile, you can use other contraceptive measures. Ask your caregiver for suggestions. Condoms and spermicidal cream are most often recommended. Don't use the pill if you are nursing, as the hormones it contains are secreted into the milk.

Note: Some obstetricians now prescribe low-dose birth-control pills for nursing mothers, since there is recent literature supporting this decision. It is important for the mother to check with her pediatrician regarding this matter. Obstetrician and pediatrician should be in agreement before the nursing mother starts taking a low-dose oral contraceptive.

Minor Problems
You may feel tender and sore when you first attempt intercourse. Feeling sore is normal even if you haven't been torn or had an episiotomy. The perineal tissues have been stretched and were probably bruised during childbirth. The woman may involuntarily tighten when her partner penetrates, increasing discomfort. She

should try to relax, while the man, of course, should be gentle. It often helps if she controls penetration by guiding the penis into the vagina.

Meanwhile, "The Blossom" exercise (see pages 99–100) will hasten healing as it restores muscle tone.

If discomfort is extreme, avoid intercourse for a while longer and consult your caregiver.

Large tears or an episiotomy preclude lovemaking until the stitches have healed (two to three weeks). Preventing or minimizing tearing and an episiotomy are discussed on pages 76–78. Even after the stitches are healed, intercourse may be uncomfortable at first. The scar tissue at the episiotomy site may be tender for a while. Soreness accompanying lovemaking may last several weeks or even longer, depending on the size of the episiotomy and the skill with which it is repaired.

The episiotomy scar is on the lower part of the vagina, either extending toward the anus or angling off to one side (depending on the type of episiotomy incision). To minimize discomfort, simply vary your lovemaking position so that pressure is away from the stitched area. The woman on top or both partners side-lying will accomplish this. Both of these positions will also avoid pressure on tender breasts.

Far from impairing postpartum recovery, intercourse actually promotes perineal healing at the site of the episiotomy.[2, 3]

Vaginal lubrication is often considerably reduced for a while as a result of hormonal changes following birth. Until ovulation resumes, the vagina may not secrete as much fluid as it did before pregnancy. Ovulation may be delayed until after the baby is partially or completely weaned.

Without the woman's natural lubricant, intercourse may be uncomfortable. If this is a problem, you can try a longer period of foreplay to encourage the vagina to moisten as much as possible naturally. Should this fail to produce sufficient lubrication, consider using a lubricant such as K-Y jelly. A couple may also try using their own saliva. Some find this more attractive than "unnatural" lubricants.

Lower sexual desire may also affect the vaginal secretions. The vagina's secretory mechanism is somewhat analogous to the man's erection. As a woman becomes more sexually aroused, the vagina moistens. However, since lower sexual desire is only one possible factor affecting vaginal secretion after birth, the man should be reassured that decreased lubrication doesn't imply that the woman is no longer attracted to him.

As much as we love to have them around, babies seem to have a way of waking up and crying just when parents are making love. Few things are more frustrating than continually interrupted lovemaking. For the sake of peace and sanity, consider putting the baby in another, nearby room. You can also put a screen of sound between you and your baby with soft music. Then you won't hear the child's every breath but will be able to hear if there is an emergency.

Overtiredness, a very common postpartum complaint, is probably the greatest detriment to lovemaking. Taking a nap—if at all possible—will make you feel more receptive to your partner. See pages 84–86 for additional suggestions on preventing or reducing fatigue.

Maternal Self-Image

Many new mothers feel unattractive after birth. Some imagine they are no longer desirable, sexual beings any more.

To many, the maternal role represents domesticity. Motherliness and all it connotes is not often associated with being a lover. But couples soon get used to the change, if in fact they notice a change in attitude at all.

In addition, the new mother's body image may be a carry-over from the way she (and her partner) thought of her changing body during pregnancy. Many expectant mothers see themselves as misshapen, awkward, and even ugly during the later prenatal months. Such a negative body image is largely a result of two factors.

First, our medicalized view of birth has given many of us an image of pregnancy as a condition bordering on illness, rather than the state of radiant health and creativity that it is. This may prevent us from fully appreciating the special beauty of the childbearing woman.

Second, in this society we tend to equate slimness with beauty. Of course, obesity is unhealthy. But the baby in the womb is no hunk of flab, nor are the other bodily changes associated with pregnancy weight gain. The pregnant woman has her own special beauty. Comparing her with the nonpregnant woman is a little like the story of the ugly duckling. One simply can't make valid aesthetic judgments comparing swans to ducks.

During the postpartum period, the mother's body is in a state of transition. The belly may look floppy for a while. Stretch marks, if there are any, may seem more significant than they are. But the belly does tone up and stretch marks do fade.

NURSING AND LOVEMAKING

Different books offer conflicting information on the way nursing influences sexual desire. This varies from suggesting that the nursing mother will resume intercourse sooner and enjoy it more, to claiming that the woman who breastfeeds will have little or no interest in sex. One postpartum guide gives such a grim picture of the nursing mother's supposedly altered sexual feelings that the reader is left believing it would be far better to bottle-feed!

Behind this conflicting information is the fact that a variety of recent studies have arrived at quite different conclusions. Some have found nursing to decrease, others to increase,[4] sexual desire. One study states that three-quarters of breastfeeding women don't notice any difference at all.[5] This implies that a variety of reactions are normal. "The varying responsiveness of nursing mothers to sexual arousal," write Elisabeth Bing and Libby Coleman in *Making Love During Pregnancy*, "is another indication that body chemistry is not the only determinant of lovemaking."[6]

The way nursing affects the mother's desire to make love varies, in fact, from woman to woman. Many notice no difference.

Many women find nursing sexually stimulating—and are surprised to discover they feel this way! Sexual sensations and accompanying vaginal lubrication are common when nursing a baby. Such a reaction may make the woman want to resume a relationship with her partner as soon as possible. Marianne, a nursing mother, said, "Sometimes nursing made me feel like I really wanted my husband to hurry up and get home from work."

After the birth of her first child via cesarean section, one mother said she found breastfeeding "mildly stimulating, but nothing like what I had read some women experience."

Jo Ellen, another first-time mother, recalls: "During the first month I found nursing very sexual and it made me feel very much alive. But that first month was like the peak of a high. The sexual feelings accompanying nursing didn't continue."

On the other hand, various factors may make the nursing mother feel less sexual desire: exhaustion, hormonal changes associated with lactation, and the fact that the mother does receive physical stimulation and satisfaction from her baby. Nursing satisfies a basic need for physical closeness and loving contact, on the part of the mother as well as her child. This may temporarily lower her sexual desire for her partner. But nursing will probably not interfere with a couple's sexual and emotional relationship unless it becomes a *substitute* for lovemaking and physical contact between the partners. The relationship is not likely to suffer unless the mother directs all her attention, love, and physical affection to the baby, leaving herself depleted and exhausted for her partner. (Of course, at first a new baby does seem to take all one's time and attention. But most couples can usually find time for one another as the weeks pass and they become more used to parenthood.)

However nursing affects the mother's sexual feelings, it need not keep a couple apart. "Whether nursing makes a woman eager for intercourse or hesitant about it," write Mary Lou Rozdilsky and Barbara Benet in their postpartum guide, *What Now?*, "if you are close as a couple there are other equally important pulls toward intimacy and intercourse. Even if nursing affects the way a woman feels sexually, it will probably not stand in the way of her sharing a full sex life."[7]

Some couples choose bottle-feeding only because they believe the mother will look more attractive if she is not nursing and leaking milk from time to time. But many new fathers, on the contrary, find themselves quite attracted to their partner while she is nursing the child.

The couple may find a change in one basic attitude. The breasts now take on a new significance. No longer are they sexual objects alone. "Previously breasts were seen as purely sexual, and uncovering them was often a portent of lovemaking; now they are utilitarian and are uncovered whenever the baby needs feeding. Switching back and forth from casual acceptance of the practical and nurturant aspects of breastfeeding, to involving the breasts in sexual foreplay, may be more of a switch than some people can make. Many men may be extremely turned on by the larger, fuller breasts of their nursing wives, and at the same time feel unsure whether it's entirely proper to be sexually excited by their baby's source of food."[8]

Though the breasts are clearly the source of the baby's food, this doesn't prevent both partners from deriving pleasure from the breasts in other ways if they so desire.

Milk may leak or even squirt from the nipples when the nursing mother is sexually excited, and particularly during orgasm. Some new fathers dislike getting milk on them. As one of my colleagues puts it, "If milk lets down during lovemaking, some men think their partner just doesn't work right any more." Arlene said of her husband, "He wouldn't touch me from the waist up. He hated getting milk on him. I couldn't get it through his head that he and the baby could share the breast—but in different ways."

Though many other men feel perfectly comfortable about the lactating breasts and don't mind occasional leaking milk, some women, on the other hand, feel awkward. As one new mother said, "I felt shy because my breasts were leaking, though it didn't seem to bother Frank."

If leaking milk bothers either of you, you can nurse the baby shortly before lovemaking so that there is less milk to leak. (The baby is also more apt to remain asleep after a feeding.) In addition, you can express milk after feeding the baby to be sure the breasts are empty. Or, you can wear a padded bra.

Some couples ignore the milk. Other fathers suck it. A friend of mine nurses the baby during lovemaking. As she expresses it, "The only time I know that the baby won't disturb us is when he's plugged in."

In any case, the milk often stops leaking after the first few weeks, when the nursing mother and baby have established a supply-and-demand pattern. Sometimes milk continues to leak as long as the mother nurses.

Provided the decision is a mutual one and both partners are accepting of the natural function of the breasts, nursing your baby can only add to your relationship. Nursing is an extension of your love for your child that will enhance, rather than diminish, your love for each other.

MAKING TIME FOR ONE ANOTHER

One of my colleagues once said, "After birth, the new parents tend to first fulfill the needs of the person who screams the loudest. Usually that's the baby."

Usually, but not always. The new parents also have needs. And the best way to make those needs known is to express them.

With a new baby in the house it is easy for the parents to let all their energies be channeled to the child. Sometimes it is easy to forget one another. Of course it is appropriate for both parents to spend much of their waking (and some of their sleeping!) time fulfilling the new baby's seemingly endless needs. But that doesn't mean a man and a woman should forget each other's equally real needs—physical, emotional, and intellectual.

If there are frustrations in a couple's relationship, it may seem easier to turn all one's affection to the new baby, drawing apart from one another. This can lead to less and less sharing of their feelings.

A destructive pattern can develop if either partner is unable to express unfulfilled needs, feelings of jealousy, resentment, isolation, or love. Some new fathers, for example, jealous of the attention their partner gives the new baby, or feeling their own needs are unfulfilled, begin spending extra time at work, show greater interest in a hobby, or perhaps begin an extramarital affair. During this critical period in a couple's changing lives, such activities channel energy away from the relationship.

The extramarital affair is not uncommon during the childbearing season. It does not necessarily indicate that a man no longer loves his partner or that he wishes to escape his responsibility to his family. Some men view the extramarital affair (perhaps unconsciously) as a way to survive the stressful period in their more important relationship at home. Others, feeling ignored at home, will turn to another woman to supply very real needs for attention and affection.

Many couples don't talk freely about their sexual feelings. But open communication about lovemaking and other aspects of their changing lives will insure that a couple's relationship is much smoother. This is particularly important if a problem seems to be developing or you and your partner seem to be drifting apart. Ignoring the problem will only encourage the condition to worsen.

With all there is to discover and learn and all there is to cope with, you may often be left wondering if you'll ever have time to be alone together. At times it may seem that your relationship will never be as it was before birth. You may even wonder what happened to the romance, to the freedom you once had before the baby came. Fatigue, fluctuating emotions, the baby's seemingly ceaseless demands, seem to be forever in the way. Eventually, however, the baby does become less demanding. You do adapt to your new roles.

One of the most important things you can do to keep your relationship sexually and emotionally smooth as you embark on this new era of your lives together is to make time for one another.

Arrange for time to be alone together. Go out for a walk, go out to dinner, *without* the baby. Spend time alone together at home as well. This may take some doing. For instance, re-arranging your schedule to meet the baby's. Having dinner at a different time, making love earlier or later, and so forth. You may simply have to decide that during a certain short period you will not be disturbed unless there seems to be a real emergency.

At first it may be necessary to budget your time so

that you will have the time to spend together in the evening. This is especially difficult if you have other children. Help around the home helps immensely. Lacking that, planning your day in advance can make a big difference.

Lovemaking after the baby is born is probably more important than ever in satisfying physical, emotional, and spiritual needs. The mother needs to know that she is still attractive to her partner, that she is not just a maternal figure, but her husband's lover. The father wants to know that he is still loved, still desired—that he is not second to their baby.

From time to time both parents need to be reassured that having a baby is not the end of romance but a new dimension in their love.

Notes

CHAPTER 1
1. Klaus, M. H., and J. H. Kennel, *Maternal-Infant Bonding: The Impact of Early Separation or Loss on Family Development* (St. Louis: The C. V. Mosby Co., 1976).
2. Barnet, C. R., et al., "Neonatal Separation: The Maternal Side of Interactional Deprivation," *Pediatrics*, Vol. 54: p. 197, 1970.
3. Klaus and Kennel, op. cit.

CHAPTER 2
1. Varney, Helen, *Nurse-Midwifery* (Boston: Blackwell Scientific Publications, 1980).
2. Pryor, Karen, *Nursing Your Baby* (New York: Pocket Books, 1975).
3. *The Womanly Art of Breastfeeding* (Franklin Park, Il: La Leche League International, 1963).
4. Eiger, Marvin S., and Sally Wendkos Olds, *The Complete Book of Breastfeeding* (New York: Bantam, 1972), p. 68.
5. Ibid. p. 19

CHAPTER 3
1. Wolfson, Randy Meyers, and Virginia DeLuca, *Couples With Children* (New York: Dembner Books, 1981).
2. Montague, Ashley, *21st Century Obstetrics Now!*, Edited by David Stewart and Lee Stewart (Marble Hill, MO: NAPSAC, Inc., 1977), p. 597.
3. Macfarlane, Aidan, *The Psychology of Childbirth* (Cambridge: Harvard University Press, 1978), p. 30.
4. Varney, Helen, op. cit. p. 353.
5. Breckenridge, Kati, and Lyn Delliquadri, *The New Mother Care* (Los Angeles: Tarcher, 1978), p. 11.
6. Jones, Carl, *Sharing Birth: A Father's Guide to Giving Support During Labor* (New York: William Morrow & Co., 1985).

CHAPTER 4
1. Fisher, Chloe, *Episiotomy and the Second Stage of Labor*, Edited by Sheila Kitzinger and Penny Simkin (Seattle: Pennypress, 1984), p. 58.
2. Ibid.

CHAPTER 6
1. Cohen, Nancy Wainer, and Lois J. Estner, *Silent Knife* (South Hadley, MA: Bergin & Garvey Publishers, 1983).
2. Banta, D., and S. Thacker, "Electronic Fetal Monitoring: Is It of Benefit?", *Birth & Family Journal* 6 (Winter 1979).
3. Haverkamp, A. D., et al., "The Evaluation of Continuous Heart Rate Monitoring in High Risk Pregnancy," *Am. J. Ob. Gyn.*, Vol. 125 (1976).
4. Donovan, Bonnie, *The Cesarean Birth Experience* (Boston: Beacon Press, 1978), p. 138.
5. *Childbirth Educator* magazine, Summer 1985.

CHAPTER 7
1. Bing, Elisabeth, and Libby Coleman, *Making Love During Pregnancy* (New York: Bantam, 1977), p. 139.

2. Reeder, Sharon J., Luigi Mastroianni, Jr., and Leonide L. Martin, *Maternity Nursing*, 14th edition (Philadelphia: J. B. Lippincott Co., 1980), p. 435.
3. Clark, A. L. and R. W. Hale, "Sex During and After Pregnancy," *AJN*, Vol. 74: p. 1430, 1974.
4. Masters, W. H., and V. E. Johnson, *Human Sexual Response* (Boston: Little, Brown & Co., 1966).
5. Kitzinger, Sheila, "Sex After the Baby Comes" (pamphlet) (Seattle: Pennypress, 1980).
6. Bing, and Coleman, op. cit. p. 150.
7. Rozdilsky, Mary Lou, and Barbara Benet, *What Now? A handbook for new parents* (New York: Charles Scribner's Sons, 1972), p. 107.
8. Wolfson, Randy Meyers, and Virginia DeLuca, *Couples with Children* (New York: Dembner Books, 1981), p. 76–77.

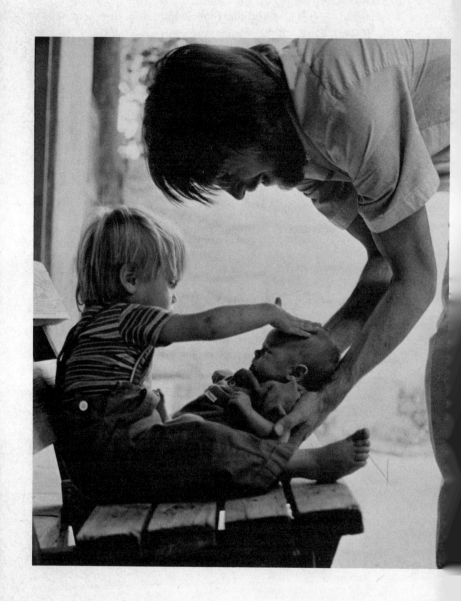

Resources

BOOKS

THE POSTPARTUM PERIOD AND PREPARING FOR PARENTHOOD

Bing, Elisabeth, and Libby Coleman, *Making Love During Pregnancy*, New York: Bantam, 1977.

Delliquadri, Lyn, and Kati Breckenridge, *The New Mother Care*, Los Angeles: Tarcher, 1978.

Harrison, Helen, and Ann Kositsky, *The Premature Baby Book: A Parent's Guide to Coping and Caring in the First Years*, New York: St. Martin's, 1984.

Jones, Carl, *Sharing Birth: A Father's Guide to Giving Support During Labor*, New York: William Morrow & Co., 1985.

Jones, Carl; Henci Goer; and Penny Simkin, "The Labor Support Guide—For Fathers, Family and Friends." (Pamphlet available from Pennypress, 1100 23rd Avenue East, Seattle, WA 98112 for $1.00.)

Klaus, Marshall, and John H. Kennell, *Bonding: The Beginnings of Parent-Infant Attachments*, New York: New American Library, 1983.

Markowitz, Elysa, and Howard Brainen, *Baby Dance: A Comprehensive Guide to Prenatal and Postpartum Exercise*, Englewood Cliffs, NJ: Prentice Hall, 1980.

Sammons, William A. and Jennifer Lewis, *Premature Babies: Different Beginning*, St. Louis: C. V. Mosby Co., 1985.

Simkin, Penny; Janet Whalley; and Ann Keppler, *Pregnancy, Childbirth and the Newborn: A Complete Guide for Expectant Parents*, Deephaven, MN: Meadowbrook, 1984.

Wolfson, Randy Meyers, and Virginia DeLuca, *Couples with Children*, New York: Dembner, 1981.

BREASTFEEDING

La Leche League, *The Womanly Art of Breastfeeding*, New York: New American Library, 1983.

Pryor, Karen, *Nursing Your Baby*, New York: Pocket Books, 1976.

FOR FATHERS

Bitman, Sam, and Sue R. Zalk, *Expectant Fathers*, New York: Ballantine, 1981.

Greenberg, Martin, M.N., *The Birth of a Father*, New York: Continuum, 1985.

Gresh, Sean, *Becoming a Father*, New York: Butterick, 1980.

Jones, Carl, *Sharing Birth: A Father's Guide to Giving Support During Labor*, New York: William Morrow & Co., 1985.

Stewart, David, "Fathering and Career: A Healthy Balance." (Booklet available from Pennypress, 1100 23rd Avenue East, Seattle, WA 98112 for $1.50.)

———, "Father to Father—On Breastfeeding," La Leche

League, 1977. (Available from La Leche League International, 9616 Minneapolis Avenue, Franklin Park, IL 60131.)

ABOUT BIRTH AND THE NEW BABY FOR CHILDREN

Anderson, Sandra VanDam, and Penny Simkin, *Birth Through Children's Eyes*, Seattle: Pennypress, 1981.

Cole, Joanna, *The New Baby at Your House*, New York: William Morrow & Co., 1985.

Malecky, M., *Mom and Dad and I Are Having a Baby*, Pennypress, 1979. (Available from Pennypress, 1100 23rd Avenue East, Seattle, WA 98112, (206)325–1419.)

POSTNATAL EXERCISE

Costanzo, Christie, *Mommy and Me Exercises: The Kidnastics Program*, Sacramento: Cougar Books, 1983.

Fienup-Riordan, Ann, *Shape Up with Baby*, Seattle: Pennypress, 1980.

Noble, Elizabeth, *Essential Exercises for the Childbearing Year*, Boston: Houghton-Mifflin, 1982.

Regnier, Susan L., *You and Me Baby: The Official YMCA Guide*, Deephaven, MN: Meadowbrook, 1984.

Whiteford, Barbara, and Margie Polden, *The Postnatal Exercise Book*, New York: Pantheon, 1984.

MULTIPLE BIRTHS

Abbe, Kathryn M., and Frances M. Gill, *Twins on Twins*, New York: Crown, 1985.

Gromada, Karen, *Mothering Multiples*, La Leche League, 1981. (Available from La Leche League International, 9616

Minneapolis Avenue, Franklin Park, IL 60131,
(312)455–7730.)

Leigh, Gillian, *All About Twins: A Handbook for Parents*, London: Routledge and Kegan, 1984.

Noble, Elizabeth, *Having Twins*, Boston: Houghton-Mifflin, 1980.

CESAREAN BIRTH

Cohen, Nancy Wainer, and Lois Estner, *Silent Knife*, South Hadley, MA: Bergin & Garvey, 1983.

Donovan, Bonnie, *The Cesarean Birth Experience*, Boston: Beacon Press, 1978.

Norwood, Christopher, *How to Avoid a Cesarean Section*, New York: Simon & Schuster, 1984.

Young, Diony, and Charles Mahan, "Unnecessary Cesareans: Ways to Avoid Them." (Pamphlet available from International Childbirth Education Association, P.O. Box 20048, Minneapolis, MN 55420.)

GRIEVING

Friedman, Rochelle, and Bonnie Gradstein, *Surviving Pregnancy Loss*, Boston: Little, Brown, 1982.

Panuthos, Claudia, *Ended Beginnings: Healing Childbearing Losses*, South Hadley, MA: Bergin & Garvey, 1984.

MISCELLANEOUS

Atlas, Stephen L., *Parents Without Partners Sourcebook*, Philadelphia: Running Press, 1984.

Brazelton, T. Berry, *Working and Caring*, Reading, MA: Addison-Wesley, 1985.

Elkins, Valmai H., *The Rights of the Pregnant Parent*, New York: Schocken Books, 1976.

Rothman, Barbara Katz, *Giving Birth: Alternatives in Childbirth* (formerly titled: *In Labor: Women and Power in the Birthplace*), New York: Penguin, 1984.

Stewart, David, *The Five Standards for Safe Childbearing*, Marble Hill, MO: NAPSAC, 1981.

PERIODICALS

American Baby

(The first six issues of this monthly magazine are sent free to expectant parents. Write to request a free six-month subscription to: American Baby Magazine, Box 13093, Boulder, CO 86322. Include your name, address, and due date.)

Mothering

This quarterly publication is available for $12 a year. Write: Mothering, P.O. Box 8410, Santa Fe, NM 87504.

All of the above books are available from the following bookstores:

- Birth and Life Bookstore, Inc.
  P. O. Box 70625
  Seattle, WA 98107
  (206)789-4444
  (Phone orders with MasterCharge, Visa, or UPS-COD accepted)

Birth and Life Bookstore also publishes *Imprints*, a quarterly review of current works about childbearing and parenthood, mailed free to customers.

- Cascade Birthing
  P. O. Box 12203
  Salem, OR 97309

(503) 378–7545

Cascade Birthing offers discounts on most of the books listed here.

- NAPSAC Bookstore
  P. O. Box 429
  Marble Hill, MO 63764
  (314)238–2010

NAPSAC also publishes a newsletter about alternatives in childbirth.

Support Groups

BREASTFEEDING

La Leche League International
9616 Minneapolis Avenue
Franklin Park, IL 60131
(312)455–7730

Provides information and support about nursing. Monthly meetings throughout the United States. Publishes many informative pamphlets. Write or call for a complete list and for the telephone number of a local La Leche League leader.

There are numerous other nursing mothers' groups throughout the country. Contact local childbirth education groups and maternity centers for names in your area.

PARENT SUPPORT GROUPS

COPE (Coping with the Overall Pregnancy/Parenting Experience)

37 Clarendon Street
Boston, MA 02116
(617)357–5588

Provides telephone support and information about support groups for parents, referrals for counseling, and information about similar support groups in different areas of the United States.

Parents' Resources
P. O. Box 107, Planetarium Station
New York, NY 10024
(212)866–4776

Provides support groups and newsletter.

CESAREAN BIRTH

C/SEC, Inc. (Cesareans/Support, Education and Concern)
22 Forest Road
Framingham, MA 01701
(617)877–8266

Provides information on cesarean birth and the options available to expectant couples.

The Cesarean Prevention Movement
P. O. Box 152, University Station
Syracuse, NY 13210
(312)424–1942

Offers information on cesarean prevention, vaginal birth after cesarean, and publishes a newsletter, *Cesarean Prevention Clarion.*

Council for Cesarean Awareness
5520 SW 92nd Avenue

Miami, FL 33165
(305)596–2699

Provides information and support regarding cesarean birth and vaginal birth after cesarean.

Cesarean Birth Council International, Inc.
P. O. Box 6081
San Jose, CA 95150
(415)343–4044

Provides information about cesarean birth and vaginal birth after cesarean, and publishes a newsletter.

COPING WITH LOSS

AMEND (Aiding a Mother Experiencing Neonatal Death)
c/o Mrs. Maureen Connelly
4324 Berrywick Terrace
St. Louis, MO 63128
(314)487–7582

Offers support and encouragement for parents who have lost a child.

The Compassionate Friends
P. O. Box 1347
Oak Brook, IL 60521
(312)323–5010

Support and encouragement for parents who have lost a child. Has chapters throughout the world. Call for a local reference.

Resolve, Inc.
P. O. Box 474
Belmont, MA 02178
(617)484–2424

Offers support for those who have experienced infertility or pregnancy loss. Call for the name of a group near you.

SHARE (A Source of Help for Airing and Resolving Experiences)
St. John's Hospital
800 East Carpenter Street
Springfield, IL 62702

Offers support to grieving parents of newborns. Has groups throughout the United States.

CHILD ABUSE

Parents Anonymous
2810 Artesia Boulevard
Redondo Beach, CA 90278
(800)352–0386 or (800)421–0353

Support over the phone, in groups, and crisis intervention for parents who abuse or are afraid they might abuse their child. Call the national office for the telephone number of a local group.

FOR ADDITIONAL RESOURCES:

Check with local hospitals, maternity centers, childbirth educators, mental health organizations, or call or write NAPSAC.

MISCELLANEOUS

Alternative Birth Crisis Coalition
P. O. Box 48371
Chicago, IL 60648
(312)625-4054

Provides referral service for both consumers and professionals involved in legal difficulties as a result of participation in a home birth. Publishes a newsletter.

American Foundation for Maternal and Child Health
30 Beekman Place
New York, NY 10022
(212)759–5510

Sponsors research, seminars, and publishes literature about unmedicated, natural birth.

NAPSAC International (The International Association of Parents & Professionals for Safe Alternatives in Childbirth)
Box 429
Marble Hill, MO 63764
(314)238–2010

Helpful information on all aspects of pregnancy, safe alternatives in childbirth, both in and out of the hospital, VBAC (vaginal birth after cesarean), breastfeeding, infant care, and childrearing. Publishes *Directory of Alternative Birth Services*, listing midwives, natural-birth oriented physicians, birth centers, family-centered hospitals, childbirth educators, breastfeeding counselors, and much more. Write for free brochure, membership information, and catalogue.

Index

Sexual relationship
  emotional and physical fac-
    tors influencing, 158–60
Shape Up with Baby (Fienup-
    Riordan), 96
SHARE, 186
*Sharing Birth: A Father's Guide to
    Giving Support During Labor*
    (Jones), 133, 135
Shoulder pain, after Cesarean,
    151
Siblings, 12, 144
Silent Knife (Cohen and Estner),
    129
Sitz baths, 79, 88
Six-week check-up (postpar-
    tum), 44
Skin pigmentation, changes in,
    31. *See also* Areola.
Spinal cord, 134
Spinal flexibility, 112, 116–
    17
Stretch marks, 31
Supplemental feeding,
    145
Support groups, 186,
    187
Surgery. *See* Cesarean.

T

Tail bone, 29
"Taking in" phase, 4
Tearing. *See* Perineum.
Temperature. *See* Fever.

Tension, 120, 121–23
Third-stage labor, 11
Trimesters, 2

U

Umbilical cord. *See* Placenta.
Urinary incontinence, 23, 29,
    91, 99
Urinary tract infection, 86, 87
Urination, 75, 86, 87, 99
    burning sensation during, 43
Uterine atony (relaxed uterus),
    24
Uterine contractions
  baby's sucking stimulates,
    147
  pitocin, 137
Uterine muscles, 11
Uterine prolapse, 99
Uterus, 11, 19, 20, 23–26, 28,
    44, 74, 75, 91, 93, 137

V

Vagina, 27, 28, 29
Vaginal birth, 127, 128, 133,
    135
Vaginal discharge, 25, 26, 137.
    See also Lochia
Vaginal lubrication, 163, 164,
    166

W

X

About the Author

A certified childbirth educator, Carl Jones is the author of *Sharing Birth: A Father's Guide to Giving Support During Labor* and co-author of the popular pamphlet, "The Labor Support Guide—For Fathers, Family and Friends." He conducts workshops for health professionals and expectant parents throughout the United States and is often a guest on radio and television shows. He lives in the Boston area with his wife, Jan, and their three sons, Carl, Paul, and Jonathan.

About the Photographer

Photographer Lyn Jones has for the past seventeen years documented the human journey through her various experiences including her work as house photographer at Cornucopia Institute, photo essayist for Judy Chicago's Dinner Party, and contributing photographer for *Mothering* magazine and numerous other publications. More recently as a birth counselor and a mother of two, she finds herself involved in yet another aspect of life . . . the birth process.